16 STEPS TO HEALTH AND ENERGY

A Program of Color & Visual Meditation, Movement & Chakra Balance

Other titles by Theo. Gimbel:

Healing Through Colour
Form, Sound, Colour And Healing
Key, Lock and Door: Healing and Meditation

Theo. Gimbel, a life-long student of the healing powers of colour, is a well-known teacher and colour healer, holding regular workshops. He has built up Hygeia College of Colour Therapy as a centre for this work, in Gloucestershire, where he lives and works. Pauline Wills has been practising and teaching yoga for more than twenty years and is also qualified as a colour therapist. Theo. and Pauline now work closely together, combining and teaching yoga and colour.

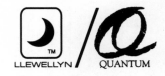

LLEWELLYN   QUANTUM

16 STEPS TO HEALTH AND ENERGY

A Program of Color & Visual Meditation,
Movement & Chakra Balance

Pauline Wills & Theo. Gimbel

1992
Llewellyn Publications
St. Paul, Minnesota 55164-0383, U.S.A.

quantum © W. Foulsham & Co. Ltd.

First U.S. Edition, 1992
First Printing, 1992

Cover art by Tom Canny

Interior photographs by Elizabeth Furth

Library of Congress Cataloging-in-Publication Data
  Wills, Pauline.
     16 steps to health and energy: a program of color & visual
  meditation, movement & chakra balance / Pauline Wills &
  Theo. Gimbel. — 1st U.S. ed.
       p.   cm.
     Includes bibliographical references and index.
     ISBN 0-87542-871-1
     1. Yoga. 2. Meditation. 3. Chakras. 4. Color—Psychological
  aspects. I. Gimbel, Theo. II. Title.
  RA781.7.W55   1992   92-2940
  613.7′046—dc   CIP

This Llewellyn/Quantum edition produced for
U.S.A. and Canada under license by:

Llewellyn Publications
A Division of Llewellyn Worldwide, Ltd.
P.O. Box 64383, St. Paul, MN 55164-0383, U.S.A.

Dedicated to my aunt, Miss Rose Grainger, for all the love, care and guidance that she has given to me over the years. My deepest thanks and gratitude.

CONTENTS

FOREWORD

My introduction to yoga was about twenty-three years ago. I was fortunate to have an Indian teacher who was devoted to the yogic way of life. Once started, I never looked back.

Studying and teaching yoga over many years I became fascinated by and deeply interested in colour. As I sought to find out more about colour and about ways in which it could be used, I was introduced to Theo. Gimbel who has spent many years researching this field. Through his research, the Hygeia College of Colour Therapy was founded. I took the course at Hygeia College and eventually qualified as a colour therapist. I was then invited by Theo. to work with him in combining and teaching yoga and colour. Some people may think this a rather unusual combination, others may view it with interest and some may already be working with it. We will show in this book how colour and yoga is not an unusual combination: they are both integral in the processes of healing and self-development that we describe.

The word yoga comes from the sanskrit word 'yuj', meaning to yoke, join or unite. The individual is a triad comprising body, mind and spirit, and the aim of yoga is to bring these three aspects into harmony, to make a person whole.

Yoga is a discipline which can become a way of life. It is believed to be one of the oldest known disciplines. It is based on the eight steps of yoga set out by the Indian sage Patanjali in his aphorisms. These eight steps are: Yamas (restraints), Niyamas (observances), Asana (posture), Pranayama (breath control), Pratyahara (sense withdrawal), Dharana (concentration), Dhyana (meditation) and Samadhi (a state of super-consciousness). Through the practice of these steps, one reaches the ultimate aim of yoga which is realisation of the true self. One can take many lifetimes to reach this goal.

In studying yoga, we learn about the subtle anatomy of the individual. We learn that we have not just a physical body but several bodies which interpenetrate. These bodies form the aura which surrounds each person. It is said that the size of the aura depends upon how evolved a person is spiritually. The aura of the Buddha is said to have extended for three miles. One of these auric bodies is the 'etheric' or energy body. In it are seven main 'chakras' or energy centres, and from these, visible to the inner eye, radiate the seven colours of the spectrum: red, orange, yellow, green, blue, indigo and violet. The violet radiating from the top chakra lifts up into magenta and then into the pure white light of God consciousness. These colours radiate out from the chakras into the aura, clothing us with a coat of many colours. The colours in the aura are continually changing, according to our physical, emotional and mental state. The darker murky shades of a colour represent the negative aspects and the bright clear shades the positive.

People with 'auric sight' claim to diagnose illness through observing the aura. Dis-ease starts in the subtle anatomy and then manifests in the physical body. Like all things manifested in the universe, colour is an energy and as such can be used to heal. Yoga is also therapeutic, so by combining the two, the benefits are increased.

In order to use colour, either in combination with yoga or by itself, one has to learn to visualise it, to sense and to feel it. To do this, the most perfect and beautiful instrument which we have, namely the human body, has to be sensitised. Each chapter of this book deals with one of the chakras. With each chakra you will find appropriate yoga asanas (postures), and a visualisation exercise which will

11

help you to feel, love, visualise and appreciate the beauty of colour. You can work with one colour for a week or with a different colour each day.

When using this book, do not spend the whole of one practice session working on just one chakra. This will over-stimulate the energy centre and may be detrimental rather than beneficial. The aim is to bring the body into balance and to do this, you should work with all of the centres, practising one or two postures from each. Ideally you should start with the crown chakra and work downwards. The reason for this is that the main energy flow is from the base chakra upwards, and to allow this energy to flow freely any blockages above it have to be cleared. Also included with our description of each chakra is the corresponding 'yantra'. A yantra is a geometrical figure whose form and content is related to the qualities of its corresponding chakra. The yantra can be used as an object for meditation.

To benefit fully from yoga and colour, you should practise for at least one hour daily: forty minutes on posture and twenty minutes on visualisation and meditation with colour. Set aside the same time each day for your practice, if this is possible. Make sure that the place you choose is quiet, well ventilated and warm, and one where you will not be disturbed.

Always practise on an empty stomach as asanas interfere with the digestion. Practise the asanas slowly and with awareness. Once you are in a posture, hold it for as long as is comfortable, unless otherwise stated. At the same time, visualise the colour which radiates from the chakra. Try to feel the effect the colour is having on you. If your mind wanders, gently bring it back. Do not be disheartened if you cannot achieve this immediately. Sometimes it can take many months of practice. If you are unable to go fully into a posture, just go as far as the body allows. With practice the body will become supple and you will be able to extend further into a posture. Remember the first law of yoga is non-violence: this includes non-violence to your own body.

At the end of your practice session, lie down, cover yourself with a blanket and relax. Play some quiet music and turn your thoughts inwards, feeling the benefits that you have gained.

Whichever path you may be following, I hope that this book opens up for you the beauty, joy and therapeutic benefits of both yoga and colour.

Pauline Wills

ACKNOWLEDGEMENTS

The authors wish to thank those who have given them so much support during the months of work on this book. Their thanks go to Patricia Jackson for proof reading, Elizabeth Furth for the photography, and yoga instructor, Reginald Money, for his help with the postures. Pauline wishes to thank Mr I.J. Patel, her own yoga master for his teaching, inspiration and guidance over the past twenty-three years. Theo. would like to express his special thanks to Pauline who introduced him to the ancient teaching of yoga and the insight which this has given him into its healing powers.

INTRODUCTION

When we are in the right place, at the right time for the right purpose, we meet up with those of a like mind, and discover the reasons for this. My meeting with Pauline Wills was such a case in point, and we soon found that colour and yoga are closely related, and that a 'conversation' between yoga and colour provided us with an unending stream of new insights. We found that when the two energies of yoga and colour meet, both can be deepened to a point which has probably never before been possible in this age. Colour-consciousness and movement-awareness change and become akin to each other. They become yoga–colour or colour–yoga. When these two beautiful energies work together as partners, they are able to promote an increased sense of well being.

May this book be a guiding thread for all those who are ready to increase their knowledge, and who are seeking a further way to health and self-awareness.

Theo. Gimbel

WORKING WITH THE WORKSHEETS

At the back of this book, after the example practice sessions, you will find a series of 16 worksheets. These have been designed from the information that is contained within the main book and can be used as the basis for individual work — you can 'mix and match' your own work programme from them — or for group workshops; each worksheet represents the work that can be practised on a single workshop. In other words the book and worksheets are suitable for teachers and students alike.

Further, on the back of each worksheet you will find an image reproduced in full colour so that you have all the material that is required for a successful combination of colour meditation and healing with the yoga exercises.

You will find that each exercise on a worksheet has been cross-referenced with the appropriate section in the main book. You can then use the main book to learn more background information to the exercises and why you are practising them, and to help you feel assured that you are performing the meditations and postures correctly.

The worksheets provide you with the means to make practical use of the book. It is advisable to work with each sheet for four to seven days before moving on to the next one. On the back of the sheets, you will find drawings of either one of the chakras or yantras, or a picture describing the meditation which has been given on the front.

It is through working with our inner being that we are able to sort out a large part of our own reactions to life. Some of the images you will want to use only for your own personal development; others can be used to develop a form of communication with friends. Perhaps some of them can help you to express your creativity through painting, poetry or even acting. This can be the means to externalising the inner awakening of your soul.

When you are working with the worksheets, please refer to the relevant pages in the book. This is important. If you find that you have a physical limitation which prevents you from practising certain postures, select a different posture which activates the same chakra and which you are able to do. Never think that you know how to go into a posture until you are experienced. Always look it up in the book.

16

The worksheets can be worked through in order, or they can be used to suit your own purposes. For example, you could work with a particular colour and then its complementary: magenta with green; violet with yellow; indigo with orange; blue with red.

You could work with magenta and green for one session or alternate these two colours in the course of a week. The same applies for the remaining colours. The possibilities are numerous and a challenge to your imagination and creativity.

We hope sincerely that all of you who work with this book may find a deeper understanding of yourself, discovering your potential for health and wholeness, realising your full potential as a spiritual as well as physical being. Through this may you find your inner peace.

LINKS BETWEEN YOGA AND COLOUR

All manifested energies, crystals, plants, animals and humans obey the laws of densification. From the immeasurable darkness state, through to the light by which the colours of the visible spectrum descend, the energies of creation progress into a density state where the colours can again no longer be seen. So believed the ancient yogis who saw the descending scales of colour as connected with the appearance of the column of the energy centres of consciousness, the chakras. The spirit energy, the almost completely white light which is transfused with a beautiful drop of red-love colour, takes on the energy of manifestation. This is also known as 'samadhi', the no-thing, because it is the absolute where all calculations cease, where no judgement can start, but which is the source of all life . . .

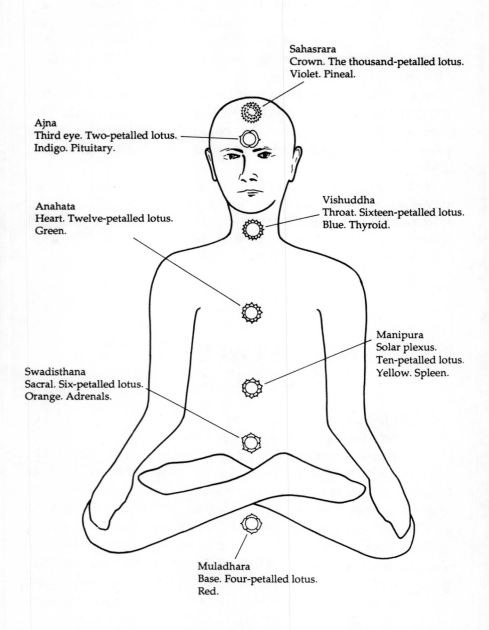

Sahasrara
Crown. The thousand-petalled lotus.
Violet. Pineal.

Ajna
Third eye. Two-petalled lotus.
Indigo. Pituitary.

Anahata
Heart. Twelve-petalled lotus.
Green.

Vishuddha
Throat. Sixteen-petalled lotus.
Blue. Thyroid.

Manipura
Solar plexus.
Ten-petalled lotus.
Yellow. Spleen.

Swadisthana
Sacral. Six-petalled lotus.
Orange. Adrenals.

Muladhara
Base. Four-petalled lotus.
Red.

*Figure 1.   The seven main chakras or energy centres, together with their
associated colours*

18

Crown Chakra

Out of this comes the colour *violet* which creates the thousand-petalled lotus flower. Although still infinite, it has its first recognition in the mental–spiritual stage. A thousand symbolises infinity. Infinity is the first concept, the crown chakra, perfection.

Third-eye Chakra

Now must arise vision, the images that can begin to bring energy into being. So the ancient, but also the now enlightened master saw in this next step of becoming, the *indigo* colour. When we wish to measure, we need two points between which we can measure. Here we have the two-petalled indigo lotus in the third eye.

Throat Chakra

Descending further into manifestation, the colour *blue* appears in the throat chakra. Here we find that the colour is represented in the form of a sixteen-petalled lotus flower. This energy centre manifests sounds and prepares the silent spaces to gather delicate matter. Sixteen is the double eight of the two octogons of harmony which overshadow each other.

Heart Chakra

On the rung below, we come to the heart, which appears in the colour *green*. This is the colour of balance upon which the scale is suspended to measure out more manifestations and energy forms. The twelve petals of its lotus indicate the time measure, the cycle of the year, the zodiac, the twelve stages of man.

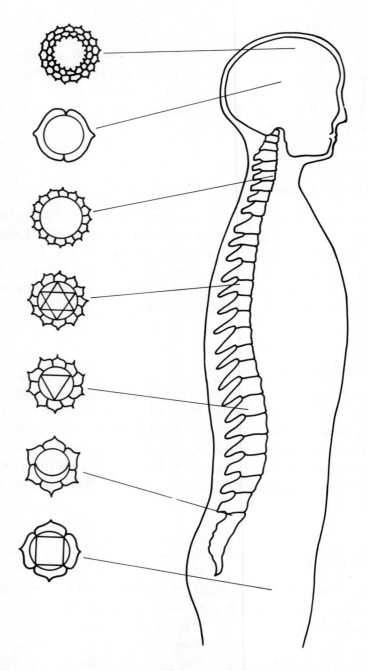

Figure 2. Position of the chakras as viewed from the side of the body

Solar-plexus Chakra

The step below is the *yellow* colour, the colour of logic and intellect. This is used to transmute the descending energies so that they can now be revealed as matter. The yellow lotus flower with ten petals represents logic and the transformation of spirit into matter.

Sacral Chakra

Now begins the joy of Eros in the *orange* colour. This colour causes the anchor to take hold of the energies with intention to create. The six petals of its orange lotus flower are the plane through which the order of manifestation will communicate with the Air, Fire, Water and Earth elements. The sacral chakra provides the images which can now create a further instrument of creation, namely the body.

Base Chakra

Only with the power of the *red* colour, which causes densification of the descending forces of life, do we now manifest in the womb of our mother. Each of these energies provides an etheric chemical change to let the embryo develop. The four petals of this lotus flower are the orientation of the heavens now made manifest on earth: north, south, east, west. Thus we are born through the colours into this life and stand here as one who can be weighed, measured and counted.

> When his mind, intellect and self are under control freed from restless desire, so that they rest in the spirit within, a man becomes a Yukta — one in communion with God. A lamp does not flicker in a place where no wind blows; so it is with a yogi, who controls his mind, intellect and self, being absorbed in the spirit within him. When the restlessness of the mind, intellect and self is stilled through the practice of yoga, the yogi by the grace of the spirit within himself finds fulfilment. Then he knows the joy eternal which is beyond the pale of the senses which his reason cannot grasp. He abides in this reality and

moves not therefrom: He has found the treasure above all others. There is nothing higher than this. He who has achieved it, shall not be moved by the greatest sorrow. This is the real meaning of yoga, a deliverance from contact with pain and sorrow.

Bhagavad Gita, Chapter 6

RELAXATION

Living in this modern world with all of its noise, problems and haste to fit all the things which have to be done into shorter and shorter periods, leaves the body in a constant state of tension. With a large majority of people, this has become the norm, and they are no longer aware of it. They have become so used to living in noise that they find silence frightening. If they find that they have a few hours to spare, they don't know what to do with them. Most people spend their leisure time either watching television or listening to pop music. To them this is relaxation. Is it? Can the body completely relax if the mind is constantly active or being bombarded with noise? These people then find that when they attempt to sleep, their minds are so active that they start to suffer from insomnia. A vicious circle then starts. Sleep is essential to the well being of the body. During this time, toxins are eliminated and healing takes place. The body and mind are re-energised in preparation for a new day. If this does not happen, when the new day dawns, they feel tired, depleted of energy and this leads to a greater degree of tension and eventually to hypertension.

Apart from daily living, there are other factors which can cause tension. Unhappy relationships, divorce, a change of job or a house move. These are but a few. Once the cause of stress has been remedied, then the tension is released. If one cannot immediately find a remedy, then one has to try and detach from the situation until it has been resolved. Frequently this detachment, not easy to practise, allows one to look in on the problem and thereby see more easily the solution.

Tension in the physical body interferes with the functioning of all its systems. This can lead to complaints such as headaches, asthma, constipation, palpitations, water retention and indigestion. If this is allowed to continue and the cause not remedied, then more serious conditions can develop such as heart attack, stomach ulcers and cancer.

If a person has lived with tension over many years, it will take time and practice to reverse this situation and to allow relaxation to become the norm. Firstly one has to become aware of the tension and then gradually learn to let go of it. When I am teaching my students relaxation, I always tell them to try to be aware of their bodies during the normal working day, to stop what they are doing several times during the day, and to feel how tense the body is, then gently to relax it. By doing this, one learns to know when the body is tense and what situations are producing this tension. This is the beginning of learning to let go and relax.

If a person is very tense, a blue light shining in a room during relaxation is a great help. Blue is the colour of expansion and helps a person to let go. Sleeping under a blue light and in blue sheets will help insomniacs. If a lot of coffee or tea is drunk and/or cigarettes smoked it is beneficial to reduce the intake of these or better still to give them up. They are all stimulants and can make the body over active.

If you have suffered from tension over many years, remember that it is not going to vanish miraculously overnight. But, if the exercises which have been given are worked with regularly, then the mind and body will become more relaxed, health will improve and a greater sense of well being will follow.

Simple Relaxation

Lie on your back on the floor in savāsana (corpse posture). Make sure that your body is straight and your chin tucked in. Your legs should be slightly apart with your hands by your sides, palms facing upwards.

Relax your mind, and visualise any thoughts as beautiful bubbles which float up into the atmosphere and then gently disperse. When your mind has become calm and peaceful, bring your concentration into your physical body. Feel each part of your body for any tension. Start with your head and work down your body to your feet. Gently let go of any tension and feel yourself starting to relax. It is much easier to go into a posture with relaxed muscles than with ones which are in tension. When you have released as much tension from your body as you can, spend a few moments in this relaxed state.

On the next inhalation, bring your arms up over your head and stretch your whole body. Exhaling, bring your arms back down to your sides. Repeat this twice more. Now gently roll over onto your side and sit up.

Relaxation Exercise No. 1

The following relaxations can be used after a session of yoga or when you are feeling tired or tense, particularly after a hard day's work. Whenever you practise relaxation, always practise in a place which is quiet and warm and where you will not be disturbed. If you find it helpful, play some soft background music which you find restful.

Lie down on your back on the floor in savāsana (corpse posture). Make sure that your body is straight. Place your hands by your side with the palms facing upwards. If you find it more comfortable, a small pillow can be placed beneath your head. Cover your body with a blanket. During relaxation, the metabolism slows down and the body's temperature drops. It is important that your body is kept warm because this aids relaxation. A cold body produces tension.

When your body is comfortable, try to let go of any problems, worries or thoughts that enter your mind. Visualise these thoughts as beautiful bubbles which float up into the atmosphere and disperse.

When your mind is calm and peaceful bring its concentration into your physical body. Feel your physical body and the floor beneath you which is supporting you. Bring your awareness down into both of your feet. Feel your toes, the tops and soles of your feet and all the muscles in your feet and toes. Feel for any tension in these muscles. Gently let go of this tension and allow your feet to become heavy and relaxed. From your feet, move your awareness up into both of your legs. Feel your ankles, your calves, shins, knees and thighs. Feel all of the muscles in your legs and consciously let go of any tension in these muscles. Let your legs become very very heavy and relaxed.

From your legs, move your awareness up into your abdomen. Go inside your abdomen. Look at and feel your pelvic girdle, the muscles which surround and support this skeletal structure and the organs which are contained within the abdominal cavity. Feel for any tension in these muscles and organs. Try to let this tension go gently so that your abdomen is able to relax.

From your abdomen, move your awareness up into your solar plexus. This part of the body contains ganglias of nerve endings and can therefore hold a great deal of tension. In many people the solar plexus chakra is frequently out of balance owing to this build up of tension and to emotional disturbances which are taking place. Being aware of this, feel the muscles and the organs which are connected with this part of the body. If you feel tension, gently try and let go of it. If you find it helpful, you can visualise this tension as a grey mist which floats away from the body and dissolves, leaving the muscles and organs relaxed and heavy.

From your solar plexus, move your awareness into your chest. Try to visualise and feel your rib cage, the muscles which support this and the organs which are contained within the chest cavity. Be aware of the slow inhalation and exhalation of the breath and the gentle, rhythmic beat of the heart. Remember that your heart is a large muscular organ and therefore is also prone to tension. Let go of any tension that you feel and let your chest become relaxed and heavy.

When you have relaxed this area as much as you are able to, bring your concentration into your shoulders, arms and hands. Starting with your shoulders and working down both of your arms into your hands and fingers, release any tension in this part of your body.

From your arms and hands, bring your concentration back into your neck and head. Feel all round your neck for tension and release it. Relax your throat. Move your awareness up into your head. Relax your jaws, your tongue, cheeks, eyes, forehead, the top and the back of your head. Feel your head becoming heavy and relaxed.

Finally, bring your awareness into the whole of your body. Mentally go over it and find any parts which are still tense. Try to release this tension. When you have done this, remain in this relaxed state for some time. Imagine the cells of your body being re-energised and re-vitalised. If you have music playing in the background, let your mind rest quietly in this music.

At the end of your relaxation time, start gently to bring the body back into everyday activity. Start to move your toes, then move your feet in tiny circles. Start to flex the muscles in your hands and move your fingers as if you are playing a piano keyboard. On the next inhalation, raise your arms over your head and stretch your whole body. Breathing out, bring your arms back to your sides. Repeat this twice more. Slowly move your head from side to side, then open your eyes. When ready, roll over onto your right side and sit up. Take note of how relaxed your body feels. Remember that the more you practise, the greater will be the depth of relaxation that you will achieve.

Relaxation Exercise No. 2

Follow the instructions given at the beginning of Relaxation No. 1.

When your body is comfortable and your mind is at peace, bring your concentration down into both of your feet. Tense up all the muscles in your feet and toes. Be conscious of what this tension is doing to your feet. Hold for about ten seconds and then let go. As the muscles in your feet relax, compare this state of relaxation to the previous one of tension.

From your feet, bring your concentration into both of your legs, from your ankles to your thighs. Tense the muscles and hold before releasing and allowing your legs to relax. Be aware of how heavy they become in relaxation.

Now move your attention up into your abdomen. Tense your abdomen. Feel how the organs inside the abdominal cavity as well as the muscles which surround it have gone into tension. Try to be aware of how this tension prevents these organs from working efficiently. After ten seconds release. Allow your abdomen to become heavy and relaxed.

Come up into your solar plexus. Again, as you tense this part of your body, be conscious that you are tensing the organs as well as the muscles. Hold and then release. Allow your solar plexus to relax. If you are normally a tense person, you may not feel such a marked difference between relaxing and tensing in this area of the body. In a tense person, this area is usually in a permanent state of tension and this becomes the norm.

Now move your attention up into your chest. Tense your chest. Notice how this tension affects your breathing and heart rhythm. Hold for five seconds and then release. As your chest relaxes, feel how much easier it is to breathe and how your heart beat slows down.

Take your awareness along your shoulders, down your arms and into your hands and fingers. Create tension in this area of your body. Hold and then relax. Feel your hands and arms becoming heavy and relaxed.

Next, bring your awareness into your neck and head. Tense the muscles in your neck, jaws, cheeks, eyes, forehead and the top and back of your head. Be conscious of how easy it is for this tension to create headaches. Hold and then release. Let your neck and head relax and become heavy.

Finally, tense every muscle and organ in your physical body. Be very aware of how this feels and what it is doing to your body. Release, and let your body go into that state of deep relaxation and heaviness. Remain in this state for a while.

At the end of this time, bring your body back into everyday activity as described at the end of Relaxation No. 1.

Relaxation Exercise No. 3

Prepare yourself for this relaxation as described at the beginning of Relaxation No. 1. Make sure that your body is warm and comfortable and that your mind is at peace.

Imagine that it is a beautifully warm and sunny day and that you are lying on the beach in a small sandy alcove, surrounded by grey cliffs which have small green rock plants growing out of their crevices. You feel the softness of the sand beneath you and its slight movement as some of the small grains trickle through your fingers. Look at the blue sky above and sense the warmth from the sun penetrating your body. Close your eyes and listen to the cry of the seagulls and the roar of the waves as they break on the shore.

Lying and listening to these sounds, you become aware of the waves breaking on the shore and very gently lapping over your feet. The water feels cold in comparison with the warmth of the sun. As the water recedes, you feel it draw out and take with it any tension that has accumulated in your feet. Your feet relax and feel heavy. The next wave breaks and gently rolls over the sand, covering your feet and legs. The coldness of the water feels invigorating. It recedes and takes your tension with it. Your legs feel re-laxed. Hearing the next wave coming and breaking on the shore, you wait for the water to touch your feet and then move over your legs, hands, lower part of your arms and abdomen. The muscles and organs in the abdomen contract slightly as they experience the coldness of the sea. The water recedes and you allow it to take your tension with it. Listening, and waiting expectantly, you prepare yourself for the next wave. It comes and covers your body up to your neck. A slight shiver goes through your body as the water comes into contact with your chest. But this is compensated by the feeling of lightness and relaxation that you experi-ence when the water has drawn out and taken with it all of your tension.

You know that the next wave will cover your entire body, but you are not afraid. Your intuition tells you that you will be able to breathe normally under this water. Wait and listen. It is coming. You embrace the water as it covers you and give to it all tension, toxins and pain that you may be experiencing, with gratitude and love. The water slowly recedes. It leaves you feeling completely relaxed and re-newed, physically, mentally and spiritually. A feeling of joy pervades you as you once more become aware of the warmth of the sun revitalising and re-energising the whole of your being.

You lie in this state for as long as you feel comfortable.

Then start to bring your body back into everyday activity, described at the end of the first relaxation exercise. Now get up and continue your day taking this feeling of peace and love with you.

SURYA NAMASKARA

SALUTE TO THE SUN

Surya namaskara, or 'salute to the sun', is a series of twelve movements. A complete round comprises these twelve movements performed twice in succession, working with each side of the body in turn. Originally, it was meant to be practised at dawn, just as the sun was rising over the horizon, acknowledging that the sun is the bringer of prana or life force, without which we cannot live. Having said this, let me add that it can be practised at any time, particularly when you are tired and feel depleted of energy.

Surya namaskara can be done purely as a series of movements to warm up the body prior to practising asanas.

However, once you add the correct breathing, it can also be used as an awareness exercise, where your concentration is brought into the physical body, making you aware of which organs, joints and muscles are being used with each movement, and how those joints and muscles move. This enables us to learn more about the beautiful temple of the body in which we live.

Finally, surya namaskara can be used as a meditation. Each movement has its own associated mantra, or sound, and when that mantra is intoned, either aloud or mentally, in combination with the slow graceful movements of the body, a wonderful sense of peace, detachment and well-being is experienced. For those who are not familiar with sanskrit, the mantras can be quite difficult to learn. I found it useful to put them onto a tape, allowing the correct time between each mantra for the movement, until I had become familiar with them. You do not have to use the sanskrit: the English translation is just as effective. I have known people who have used the Lord's prayer as a mantra, intoning one phrase of the prayer for each movement. For example: 'Our Father' would be intoned with position one; 'Which art in heaven' with position two, and so on.

The chakra that is activated by a particular movement also radiates a colour. Look at the descriptions of the chakras given on pages 19–21 to find the appropriate colours. Instead of using a sound, or mantra, you can concentrate on the chakra and visualise its pure clear colour being poured out into your aura. But remember that visualisation of the colours is only used when you are working with surya namaskara as a meditation technique.

Surya namaskara works with every muscle in the body, removing tension, strengthening and making them supple. It also makes the spine supple, thereby helping to eliminate back problems, and tone the spinal nerves. Because it activates the chakras it also works on the endocrine glands, bringing harmony and balance to all the systems of the body. The slow and deep inhalation and exhalation of the breathing pattern rids the lungs of impurities and brings about a deep relaxation of mind and body. The circulatory system is invigorated and the organs of the body stretched and compressed, ensuring their correct functioning.

To experience the full benefits of surya namaskara, it should be practised every day, starting with three positions and slowly working up to twelve.

1st Position — PRANAMASANA — Prayer Pose

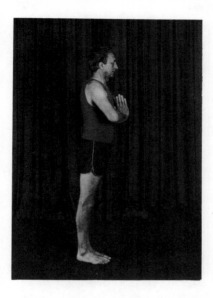

Stand in an upright position with the feet together, spine straight, shoulders back and chest expanded. Bring the hands together into the prayer position with the thumbs pointing towards the anahata or heart chakra. This is acknowledgement of the seat of the true self. Relax the whole body, breathing normally. Bring your concentration into the heart chakra. Either visualise the colour green radiating out from the chakra into the aura, or intone a mantra. The sanskrit mantra is:

OM MITRAYA NAMAHA

(Salutations to the friend of all)

2nd Position — HASTA UTTANASANA — Salutation

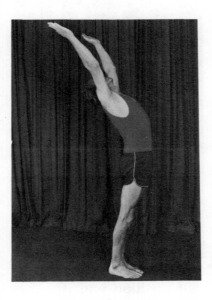

Breathing in, raise both arms frontwards over the head, keeping them straight and in line with the shoulders. Bend the trunk of the body and the head backwards. Concentrate on the vishuddhi or throat chakra. Visualise either the colour blue radiating out from the chakra into the aura, or intone a mantra. The sanskrit mantra is:

OM RAVAYE NAMAHA

(Salutations to the shining one)

3rd Position — PADANGUSTHASANA — Hand to Foot Pose

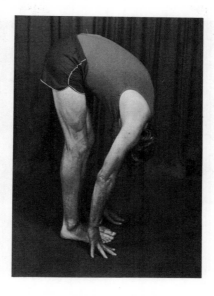

Exhaling, extend the body forward from the hips, keeping the spine straight, until the trunk of the body rests against the legs. Bring the palms of the hands onto the floor by the side of the feet, fingers facing forwards. Concentrate on swadhisthana chakra. Either visualise the colour orange radiating from the chakra into the aura, or intone a mantra. The sanskrit mantra is:

OM SURYAYA NAMAHA

(Salutations to the one who induces activity)

4th Position — ASHWA SANCHALANASANA
— Equestrian Pose

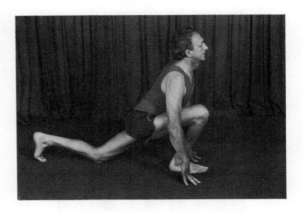

Keeping the left foot and the hands in the same position, inhale while you stretch the right leg back as far as possible, keeping the toes tucked under. At the same time bend the left leg, keeping the knee in line with the ankle. Now bend the right knee onto the floor. Lift the trunk off the left leg and raise the palms of the hands off the floor until just the fingertips are touching it. Take the head back. Concentrate on the ajna chakra. Either visualise the colour indigo radiating from the chakra out into the aura, or intone a mantra. The sanskrit mantra is:

OM BHANAVE NAMAHA

(Salutations to the one who illumines)

5th Position — ADHO MUKHA SVANASANA — Dog Pose

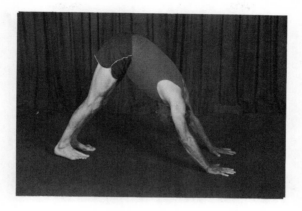

Lower the trunk back onto the left leg, letting the palms of the hands rest on the floor. Exhale while straightening the left leg and, at the same time, lift the right knee off the floor. Take the left foot back until it is in line with the right foot. Raise the buttocks in the air and lower the head between the arms, bringing it as near to the floor as possible. The arms and legs should be kept straight and the heels in contact with the ground. Concentrate on swadhisthana chakra. Either visualise the colour orange radiating from the chakra into the aura, or intone a mantra. The sanskrit mantra is:

OM KHAGAYA NAMAHA

(Salutations to the one who moves quickly in the sky)

6th Position — ASHTANGA NAMASKARA — Salute with Eight Limbs

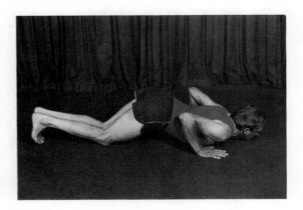

Holding the breath out, lower the body onto the floor until the toes of both feet, the knees, the chest, two hands and the chin touch the floor. The hands should be level with the chest, the hips and abdomen raised from the floor. In this posture eight parts of the body are touching the floor. This represents the eight steps of yoga described on pages 10–11. In this posture you can concentrate on manipura chakra or contemplate these steps whilst doing shallow breathing. Alternatively, visualise the colour yellow radiating from the chakra into the aura, or intone a mantra. The sanskrit mantra is:

OM PUSHNE NAMAHE

(Salutations to the giver of strength)

7th Position — BHUJANGASANA — Cobra Pose

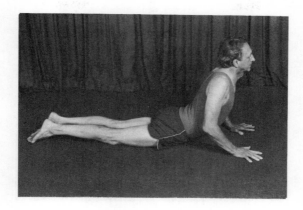

Inhaling, let the legs slide back until they are straight on the floor. Press down with the hands and raise the trunk off the floor, taking the head back. Make sure that the pubis is still in contact with the floor and that the shoulders are lowered and taken back to expand the chest. Concentrate on swadisthana chakra. Either visualise the colour orange radiating out from the chakra into the aura, or intone a mantra. The sanskrit mantra is:

OM HIRANYA GARBHAYA NAMAHA

(Salutations to the golden cosmic self)

8th Position — ADHO MUKHA SVANASANA — Dog Pose

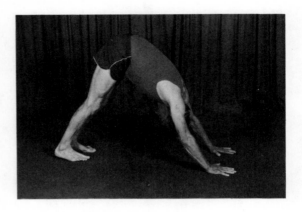

With the toes tucked under, exhale and press down with the hands and feet, raising the body off the floor, back into the dog posture. This is the same as position five on page 37. Concentrate on swadisthana chakra. Either visualise the colour orange radiating from the chakra into the aura, or intone a mantra. The sanskrit mantra is:

OM MARICHAYE NAMAHA

(Salutations to the lord of the dawn)

9th Position — ASHWA SANCHALANASANA — Equestrian Pose

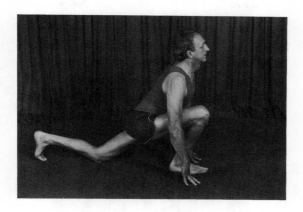

Inhaling, bend the left knee, bringing the foot between the hands. At the same time bend the right knee onto the floor. This is the same as position four on page 36. Concentrate on ajna chakra. Either visualise the colour indigo radiating out from this chakra into the aura, or intone a mantra. The sanskrit mantra is:

OM ADITYAYA NAMAHA

(Salutations to the son of Aditi)

Aditi is one of the names of the infinite cosmic mother.

10th Position — PADANGUSTHASANA — Hand-to-Foot Pose

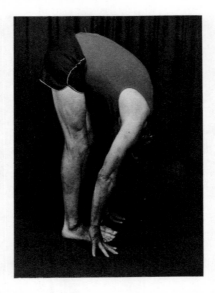

Exhaling, straighten the left leg and bring the right foot next to the left foot. Keep the palms of the hands on the floor by the side of the feet, and the trunk and head as close to the legs as possible, making sure that the spine is kept straight. This is the same as position three on page 35. Concentrate on swadisthana chakra. Either visualise the colour orange radiating out from the chakra into the aura, or intone a mantra. The sanskrit mantra is:

OM SAVITRE NAMAHA

(Salutations to the benevolent mother)

11th Position — HASTA UTTANASANA — Salutation

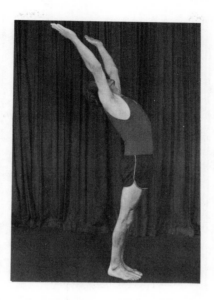

Inhaling, bring the body back to a standing posture and take the arms forwards over the head, slightly bending the trunk and taking the head back. This is the same as position two on page 34. Make sure that the feet are in line with each other. Concentrate on vishuddhi chakra. Either visualise the colour blue radiating out from the chakra into the aura, or intone a mantra. The sanskrit mantra is:

OM ARKAYA NAMAHA

(Salutations to him who is fit to be praised)

12th Position — PRANAMASANA
— Prayer Pose

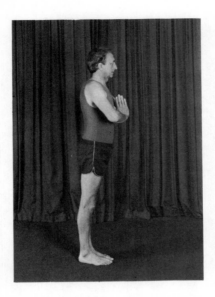

Exhaling, bring the arms down to the prayer position, with the thumbs pointing towards anahata chakra. Make sure that the feet are together and the spine straight. This is the same as position one on page 33. Concentrate on anahata chakra. Either visualise the colour green radiating out from the chakra into the aura, or intone a mantra. The sanskrit mantra is:

OM BHASKARAYA NAMAHA

(Salutations to the one who leads to enlightenment)

THE MULADHARA CHAKRA OR BASE CENTRE

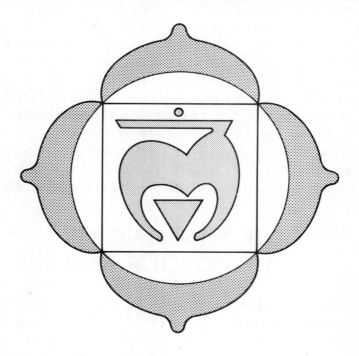

Look to this day
for it is life
the very life of life.
In its brief course lie all
the realities and truths of existence,
the joy of growth,
the splendour of action,
the glory of power.
For yesterday is but a memory.
And tomorrow is only a vision.

But today well lived
makes every yesterday a memory of happiness
and every tomorrow a vision of hope.
Look well, therefore, to this day.

Ancient Sanskrit Poem

The muladhara chakra is known as the base centre. It is symbolised by a deep red lotus with four petals. In the centre of the lotus is a yellow square. In the square is a red triangle with its apex pointing downwards. The triangle rides on an elephant with seven trunks. This is not normally shown in diagrams of the chakra, but symbolises the stability and solidarity of the earth. The presiding deities are Brahma, the creator of the universe, and Dakini the goddess, who is the controller of the skin element of the body. In the yellow square is also written the sanskrit for the mantra which is LAM. This centre contains the primal energy which is the Kundalini Shakti. It is associated with the element of Earth and regulates the sense of smell.

THE MEANING OF
THE COLOUR RED

Red is the colour that represents the present, the here and now, physical energy. It is the power of life and the Father who bestows this power. With red we are entering the central force. It is connected with sexuality, it heightens blood pressure and encourages inhalation. In its negative form it raises adrenalin and causes defensiveness, aggression and violence. The saying 'It makes me see red', indicates the aggressive aspect of this colour. There are shades of red which cover the whole range from negative to positive, from hate to love. The quality of the red which is at the centre of this range, is a power which can flow in two directions. If you look at the illustration on page 47 starting on the left side with pure love, you will see that this can descend into black–red, but that black–red can again be lifted into pure love.

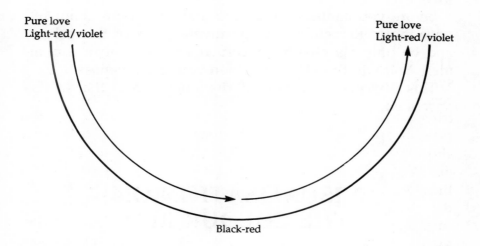

Pure love
Light-red/violet

Pure love
Light-red/violet

Black-red

Positive Red

Light-red/violet represents pure love which is selfless. To show respect for one whom you love, you give a red–violet rose.
Rose-red is admiration and personal love.
Red–orange stands for enthusiasm, joy and fun.

Negative Red

Pure red has an objective power and represents the Father.
Red–Red, still represents the Father but is seen by those who still live in fear of Him.
Intense red stands for the use of force through anger or represents taking a powertrip through someone or something.
Red–black represents Sataniel, the angel of Challenge. It denotes power over others, signifying a dictator or manipulator.

The symbol of the red chakra has four petals, representing orientation on earth: north, south, east and west. The red elephant, often in chains, is not yet free to use the red of love.

Before you continue, read the first paragraph about red once more. Remember the positive aspects of this colour, and be only marginally concerned with its negative qualities. You will thereby strengthen your positiveness.

This advice is relevant to all the other colours that will be described.

VISUALISATION ON THE COLOUR RED

Find a red flower and put it into water. Sit down in a comfortable position, placing the flower in front of you. Look at the flower. Take it into your hands and observe how delicate and perfectly shaped the petals are. Look for the varying shades of red within that flower, and notice the differences in the formation of each petal. Now gently hold the flower, placing it on the palm of your left hand. Hold the palm of your right hand about three to four inches above it. Close your eyes and bring the whole of your concentration into your hands. Try and feel through your hands the vibration of the colour. Now return the flower to its receptacle and look at it. Close your eyes and try to visualise it. Visualise the shape and the colour. Try to feel and become one with that colour. If any part of your body feels cold, visualise the colour red in that area of the body. Feel the cold being replaced by warmth. Now take this colour into the base chakra. Feel this energy centre being brought into balance, and at the same time feel the colour earthing and grounding you. Gently open your eyes and allow a few moments of reflection before ending your visualisation.

MULADHARA YANTRA

A yantra is a geometric form which is used for concentration and visualisation. The yantras are taken from the geometric forms of the chakras and are used whilst holding a posture relating to that particular energy centre. They can also be used purely for visualisation or for meditating upon.

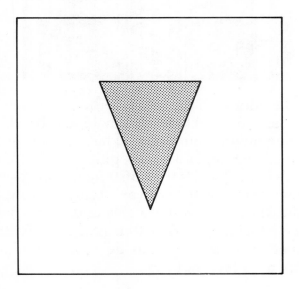

ASANAS WHICH ACTIVATE MULADHARA

Whilst holding the postures given in this book, firstly bring your awareness into the physical body, feeling which muscles are being used and which organs of the body are being stretched or compressed. Then bring that awareness into the relevant chakra and either visualise the yantra in that chakra, or the colour radiating out from the chakra into the aura bringing about balance and harmony.

The Knee Lock

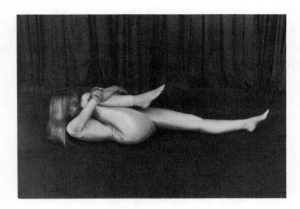

Lie flat on the floor with the legs together, hands by the side of the body and neck extended. Inhale and bend the right knee, clasping it with your arms. Exhale and bring the head as near to the knee as possible, keeping the outstretched leg in contact with the floor. If the outstretched leg loses contact with the floor, it means that you are trying to bring the head closer to the knee than you are able and compensating for this by raising this leg. Work both legs separately, then both legs together. This posture can be repeated four to five times. Relax for a few minutes.

Ardha Navasana 1 — The boat

Sit on the floor with the legs stretched out in front, keeping the spine straight. Place the palms of the hands on the floor by the hips with the fingers pointing towards the feet. Exhale and recline the trunk slightly back, simultaneously raising the legs from the floor to an angle of 60 to 65 degrees. The legs should be higher than the head and remain straight with the knees locked. Stretch the arms forward, keeping them parallel to the floor and near the thighs. If possible,

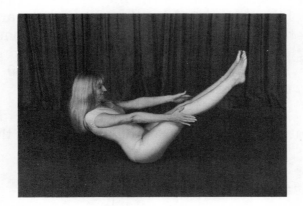

hold this posture for 30 seconds. Exhaling, come back to a sitting posture.

Benefits.   This asana reduces fat around the waistline and tones the kidneys, gall bladder, liver and spleen. It works on the thighs and abdominal muscles. It also improves balance, reduces nervous tension and aids poor digestion.

Ardha Navasana 2

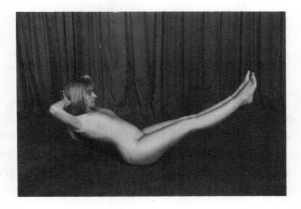

Sit on the floor with the legs stretched out in front. Keeping the spine straight, interlock the fingers and place them on the back of the head just above the neck. Exhale, and recline the trunk back simultaneously raising the legs from the floor to an angle of 30 to 35 degrees. The head should be in line with the feet. Hold this posture for about 30 seconds. Exhaling, come back to a sitting posture.

Benefits. This asana has the same benefits as ardha nava-sana 1 but has a greater strengthening effect on the back.

Garudasana — The eagle

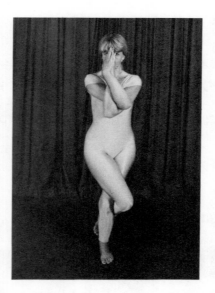

Stand in an upright posture with the toes in line, feet together and hands by your sides. Bend the right knee. Bring the left leg over the right thigh above the knee and rest the back of the left thigh on the front of the right thigh, moving the left foot behind the right calf. Gain your sense of balance in this posture. Then bend the elbows and entwine the arms so that the right elbow is resting on the front of the left upper arm near to the elbow joint. Move the right hand back to the right, and the left hand back to the left and join the palms.

Benefits. This posture strengthens the knees and ankles and removes stiffness in the shoulders. It is recommended for preventing cramp in the calf muscles. It improves balance and helps sterility and sexual debility.

The Arm–Leg Link

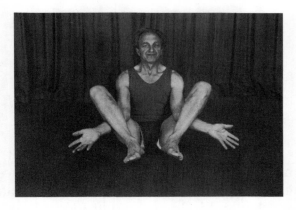

Sit on the floor with the legs stretched out in front and the spine straight. Bend the knees, placing the soles of the feet by the buttocks. The feet are about fifteen centimetres apart. Take the arms between the legs and under the knees. Exhale, and recline the trunk slightly backwards so that the feet are raised from the floor and you are balancing on the buttocks. Open the knees out as far as possible. Make sure that the spine is kept straight throughout. Hold for as long as is comfortable. Exhale, and return to the sitting position.

Benefits. This posture stretches the inner thigh muscles and is therefore a good posture to use in pregnancy. It aids balance and poise and helps in working towards the full lotus.

Padmasana — The full lotus

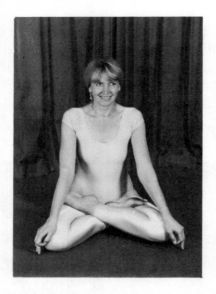

Sit on the floor with the legs straight out in front. Bend the right leg at the knee and, holding the foot, place it at the root of the left thigh so that the heel is near the navel. Now bend the left leg and holding the left foot, place it over the root of the right thigh again bringing the heel near to the navel. The soles of the feet should be turned up. This posture should be worked at slowly.

Benefits. Once this posture has been mastered, it is a relaxing pose and excellent for meditation. It tones the coccygeal and sacral nerves by supplying them with an extra flow of blood. It can help with many nervous and emotional problems. This asana directs the correct flow of prana from the base to the crown chakra.

Caution. This posture should not be practised if suffering from sciatica.

Yoga Mudrasana

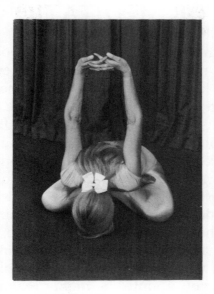

Sit in padmasana (full lotus), making sure that the spine is straight. Inhaling, clasp the hands behind the back. Exhaling, and keeping the spine straight, move the trunk forward from the hips until the chin touches the floor. At the same time raise the arms upwards. For those who are unable to sit in full lotus, this posture can be done in half lotus or in simple cross leg posture.

Benefits. This posture removes stiffness from the arms and shoulders. It intensifies the peristaltic action and relieves constipation. It improves the digestion.

Caution. If suffering from sciatica, this posture should not be attempted in full lotus.

IMPORTANT GUIDELINES
FOR MEDITATION

When using the meditations in this book, either read through them until you have retained the general outline or put them onto tape. Do not try to learn them by heart. In using your own words, you can experience the freedom to be yourself. This also enhances relaxation. In creating your own images, you will become sensitive to the energies of the colours and receive the healing that they offer you.

When you prepare yourself for meditation, find a place which is comfortable, warm and quiet, and where you will not be disturbed. You can either sit on a chair, or kneel or sit on the floor. Whichever position you choose, make sure that your spine is straight. Visualise your spine as a golden column of light which anchors you to this planet earth, but which also lifts you up into the higher realms of consciousness. You can repeat to yourself. 'I am in the right place, at the right time for the right purpose. I bless, I thank and I love.' It is a good idea at this point to prepare for the unexpected. No matter how quiet and peaceful the environment which you have chosen, unforseen things do happen, like a person walking into the room where you are and perhaps speaking to you or touching you. A sudden loud noise, or the door bell or telephone may ring. If you are unprepared for these things they can cause a shock to the physical body. Having said this, should something happen that you are not prepared for, look upon it as a teaching. Next, place yourself in a blue or golden orb of protection. Work with both of these colours in order to find out which one you feel most comfortable with.

Now start to let go of any tension in your body. Start with your feet and slowly work up towards your head. If it helps, you can visualise this tension as a grey mist which floats away from the body and is dissolved back into the elements of Earth, Water, Fire, Air and Ether. By doing this, we bless the earth because we have allowed these elements to pass through us, and then to be returned to the earth.

From your body, bring your concentration into your breathing. Let yourself become sensitive to the slow inhalation and exhalation of the breath. With each exhalation, experience your body going deeper into relaxation and your mind becoming very quiet and still. When you have reached a state of peace and tranquillity, proceed with the meditation which you have chosen.

After each meditation, you must return to the environment in which your higher self has placed you. In order to come back, you have to let go of this experience. Start to increase your inhalation and exhalation, and become aware of your physical body and the room in which you are sitting. Take a circle of light which contains a cross of light and use this symbol as a golden key to lock securely all of your chakras, which are doors to a higher perception. Start with the crown and work downwards to the brow, the throat, the heart, solar plexus, sacral, and lastly the base chakra. Having closed these doors, gently open your eyes and be completely returned to planet earth.

MEDITATION WITH THE COLOUR RED

Before starting this meditation, read the guidelines which you will find on page 56.

It is not advisable to start meditating on the colour of red if you have not had any experience in meditation. Red is a powerful colour and self-preparation is needed through the use of other meditations. If you are a beginner, read through this meditation, but do not practise it until you have been working with this book for a while.

The flame of life is covered with the colour of turquoise. This colour is brought about by the green of the leaves and the blue of the air and it causes the cooling of this red flame. The veils to this flame are carefully drawn, but we know that this flame of red is safely behind them.

Feel that you are sitting in a glade, where everything is calm and peaceful. Allow this colour of green to bring the whole of your being into balance. See before you a curtain of yellow. This colour gives you a sense of detachment, making your thoughts clear and free. Slowly draw this veil aside and you will find that a curtain of orange has been revealed to you. Allow yourself to step into this colour. Feel the anticipation of joy as this colour prepares you and gives you the respect which is needed for the power of the red colour.

Cool, balanced, detached and joyful, carefully draw aside this veil. As it falls away, you see before you the fire, the fire of life. Slowly approach and stand before this red flame of life energy. You have no need for defences, because the flame of red sings a sound, a sound of love, the love to be in the presence of pure love. You have been taken to your origin and reminded that your mother stands as the representative of Her, the spirit Mother. All the love that you are and will be streams through her heart.

You are reminded of your father. He, being the representative of Him, the Father in heaven. At this moment you are experiencing your own conception and have only the highest thoughts of pure love. You forgive both of your parents any short comings that they may have had. You also forgive yourself for your own weaknesses.

At this moment, the red flame becomes bright and pure. Bow down before it with gratitude and realise in your heart, that this red energy of love has purified all your past experiences. Reverently step back and start slowly to draw the veils back across the flame. Firstly the orange, then the yellow and finally the green veil. Turning round, you face once more the turquoise of tranquillity and peace. Amen.

THE SWADISTHANA
CHAKRA OR
SACRAL CENTRE

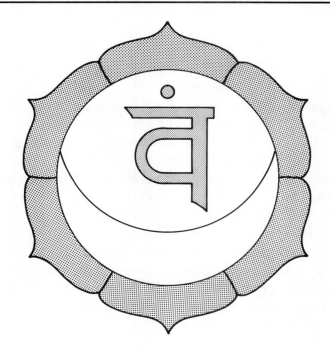

Joy

O let us live in joy, in love amongst those who hate.
Among men who hate, let us live in love.
O let us live in joy, in health amongst those who are ill.
Among men who are ill, let us live in health.

O let us live in joy, in peace amongst those who struggle.
Among men who struggle, let us live in peace.

O let us live in joy, although having nothing.
In joy let us live like spirits of light.

Health is the greatest possession, Contentment
is the greatest treasure. Confidence is the
greatest friend. Nirvana is the greatest joy.

When a man knows the solitude of silence, and
feels the joy of quietness, he is then free
from fear and sin and he feels the joy of the
Dhamma,

If you find a man who is constant, awake to the
inner light, learned, long-suffering, endowed
with devotion, a noble man, follow this good
and great man even as the moon follows the path
of the stars.

from *The Dhammapada*

The literal meaning of the word swadisthana is 'one's own abode'. This chakra is symbolised by an orange lotus flower with six petals. In its centre is a white crescent moon. The mantra is WAM. The moon and the sanskrit symbol for the mantra, ride on a crocodile which represents the Water element. The presiding deities are Lord Vishnu, the maintainer and preserver of the universe, and the goddess Rakini, controller of blood in the body. On the physical level, swadisthana is mainly associated with the organs of excretion and reproduction. Vitalisation of this centre can therefore rectify any disorders in these functions. On a deeper level, this chakra is the seat of the unconcious mind, the collective unconciousness. It is the centre of our most primitive and deep-rooted instincts. By purifying this centre, one can rise above the animal nature.

THE MEANING OF
THE COLOUR ORANGE

Orange is the colour of joy and happiness. It enables us to find the balance between the physical and mental bodies. It gives freedom to thoughts and feelings, dispersing any heaviness, and it allows the body natural joyful movements.

60

This colour enables us to respond to happiness without a feeling of guilt.

In healing, orange brings about changes in the biochemical field, and this results in the lifting of depression. It is, therefore, a good colour to use for people who are depressed. In the aura, the colour appears in the area of the lower abdomen, and according to its strength and vitality, supports life and sexual energy, and also gives joy.

In its negative form, orange can be a dominating colour, and one can feel a compulsion to remain in it, even if it is no longer necessary. If a person is placed into orange by others, it will ultimately weaken and undermine the will to the extent that the person no longer questions what he or she is doing. That person loses self-responsibility and finally becomes subservient. It can, therefore, be used to manipulate others, especially if they are not aware of its power.

VISUALISATION ON THE COLOUR ORANGE

For this visualisation and awareness exercise you should use a piece of carnelian. Carnelian is deep orange in colour and part of the agate family. It is a stone connected with the earth and its energies. Because of its connection with the earth, it stimulates a deeper love and appreciation of the beauty and gifts of the earth. Also, it can be used to ground our earth energies.

Find a place which is quiet and warm, where you will not be disturbed. Sit down in a comfortable position. Take the piece of carnelian in your left hand and close your hand over it. Close your eyes. Try to rid your mind of all unnecessary thoughts so that it becomes calm and concentrated. Bring your mind into your physical body. Go over the body, relaxing any part which is tense.

Now bring your concentration into your left hand. Firstly, try to feel the colour of the stone. Now ask that stone to allow you to feel its energies. At this point you may get pictures coming into your mind, showing you where the stone originated from. On the other hand you may not feel or see anything. Do not worry if this happens. Awareness and sensitivity are only gained by regular practice.

After ten to fifteen minutes of quietly sitting and concentrating on the stone, take it and place it against the swadisthana chakra. Try to feel it energising this centre, ridding it of any blockages. Then gently open your eyes and, before ending this exercise, allow yourself a few moments of reflection on anything that you may have experienced.

When using stones for awareness and visualisation practice, it is beneficial to cleanse them before further use. Stones are sensitive to energy fields, and the carnelian will have picked up your vibrations. The easiest way to cleanse a stone is to put it into salt water for twelve hours, preferably in the sun.

SWADISTHANA YANTRA

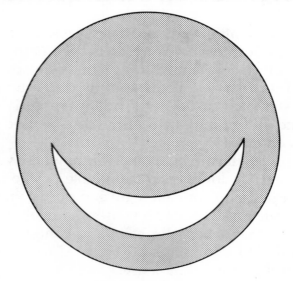

ASANAS WHICH ACTIVATE SWADISTHANA

Paschimottanasana — The back stretching posture

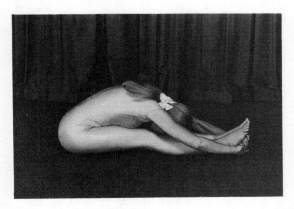

Sit on the floor with the legs extended in front of the body. Inhaling, straighten the spine and take the hands down to the feet. (If you are unable to touch your feet, place a belt round them holding either end of the belt with your hands.) Keeping the spine straight and the knees locked, exhale and slowly lower the body until it is lying flat along the legs. Hold this posture for as long as is comfortable. Inhale and come back to the sitting posture.

Benefits. This posture stretches the ham-string muscles and loosens the hip joints. It removes excess fat in the abdominal region. It tones the abdominal organs and relieves diabetes. It activates the kidneys, liver, pancreas and adrenal glands. It tones the pelvic organs and is therefore useful for eliminating sexual problems. It encourages a good flow of blood to the spinal nerves and muscles. This is a powerful asana for spiritual awakening.

Caution. This posture should not be practised by people with a slipped disc, sciatica, or chronic arthritis.

Janu Sirsasana — The head-to-knee posture

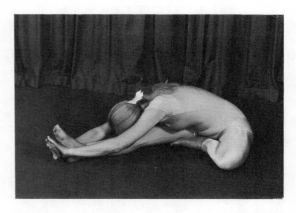

Sit on the floor with the legs extended in front of the body. Bend the right knee and place the sole of the right foot against the thigh of the left leg. (If your knee does not touch the floor, support it with a cushion or a blanket.) Inhaling, straighten the spine and extend both the hands to hold the left foot. (If you cannot reach your foot, use a belt as in the previous posture.) Exhaling, and keeping the spine straight, gently lower the body onto the left leg, making sure that the knee is kept locked. Hold for as long as is comfortable, then on an inhalation raise the body back to the sitting posture. Repeat on the other side. When the body becomes supple, the foot of the bent leg can be placed on the thigh of the outstretched leg (half lotus posture). This should not be attempted until the bent knee touches the floor.

Benefits and Caution.   These are the same as for paschimottanasana.

Upavistha Konasana — The angle posture

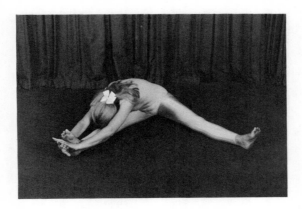

Sit on the floor with the legs spread as wide as possible. Raise the arms over the head, keeping them straight, and clasp the hands. Turn the body towards the right leg. On an inhalation, lift the body, thus straightening the spine. Whilst exhaling, gently lower the body onto the right leg keeping the knee locked and making sure that the left buttock does not lose contact with the floor. On the next inhalation, raise the body back to sitting posture. Turn the body towards the left leg and, whilst exhaling, lower the body down onto the left leg. Inhale and raise the body. On the next exhalation lower the body between the legs until it touches the floor. Inhale, whilst raising the body to sitting posture and bring the legs together. Each of these positions can be held for as long as is comfortable.

Benefits. This posture stretches the hamstring muscles and helps the blood to circulate in the pelvic region. It prevents the development of hernia and it can cure mild cases of this. It relieves sciatic pains, regularises menstruation and stimulates the ovaries.

Padangusthasana — Hand-to-foot posture

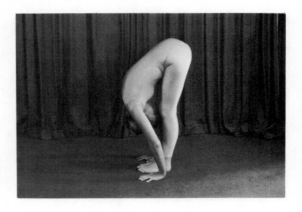

In standing posture, make sure that the spine is straight. Place the feet about fifteen centimetres apart, making sure that they are parallel and the toes of the left and right foot are in line. On an inhalation, lift up the spine; exhaling, bend the trunk forward from the hips, keeping the spine straight and the knees locked, and hold the big toes with the hands. Inhale whilst holding this position. On the next exhalation continue to lower the body onto the legs. Hold for as long as is comfortable. Inhaling, raise the body back to standing posture. (If you are unable to touch your toes, place a wooden block or pile of books in front of your feet to place your hands on.)

Benefits. This posture removes excess fat, eliminates flatulence, constipation and indigestion. It makes the spine and back muscles supple. All the spinal nerves are stimulated and toned and the metabolism is increased. It influences the reproductive system, removing sexual ailments. It gives a good flow of blood to the brain and face.

66

Caution. Not to be practised by people with back ailments or sciatica.

Supta Vajrasana — The thunderbolt

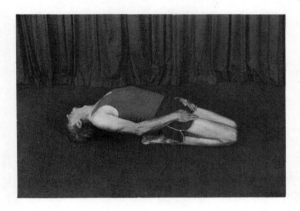

This posture also activates the vishuddhi chakra.
Kneel on the floor with the legs together and the big toes crossed. Lower the buttocks to the insides of the feet, placing the heels at the sides of the hips. Exhaling, bend the trunk backwards, supporting the body on the arms and elbows, until the head touches the ground with the back fully arched. Take the elbows off the floor and place the hands on the thighs, making sure that the knees stay together and on the ground. Hold this posture for as long as is comfortable. For those who have difficulty with this posture, the knees can be separated until the thigh muscles and spine are supple enough for the knees to be brought together. Alternatively, a blanket or blankets can be placed under the head until the spine becomes supple enough to allow the head to touch the floor.

Benefits. This posture is good for abdominal ailments, especially constipation. It tones the spinal nerves and benefits the thyroid and parathyroids. It also tones the thigh muscles and works on the knees.

67

Supta Virasana

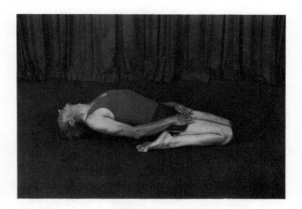

This posture also activates the vishuddhi chakra.

Kneel on the floor with the legs apart but the knees together. Lower the buttocks onto the floor between the legs. Supporting the body on the arms and elbows, arch the back backwards until the head touches the floor. Place the hands on the thighs, making sure that the knees stay together and in contact with the floor. (If you have difficulty sitting between your legs, sit on a blanket or cushions until you become supple enough to sit on the floor. If you are sitting on a cushion or blanket, you may find it necessary to place a folded blanket under your head.)

Benefits.   This posture has the same benefits as supta vajrasana, but with a greater stretching and toning of the thigh muscles.

Salabhasana — The locust

Lie on the stomach with the chin resting on the floor and the hands clasped under the thighs. Stretch the legs and tense the arms. Inhale and, holding the breath in, raise the legs and abdomen as high off the ground as possible. Exhale, and lower the legs onto the floor.

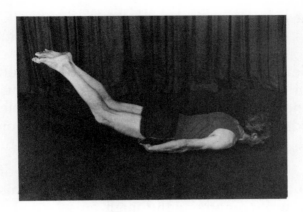

Benefits. This asana tones the liver and other abdominal organs, especially the pancreas, intestines and kidneys. The bladder and prostate gland also benefit. It stimulates the appetite and relieves and eliminates diseases of the stomach and bowels. It strengthens the lower spine and abdominal muscles and tones the sciatic nerves.

Caution. Not to be practised by people suffering from a peptic ulcer or a hernia.

Ardha Salabhasana — Half locust

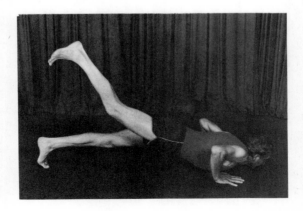

Lie on the stomach with the chin resting on the floor. Place the palms of the hands on the floor by the chest, with the fingers pointing towards the head. Tuck the toes of the left foot under. Press down on the toes of the left foot to straighten the leg and to raise it slightly off the ground. Inhale, and raise the right leg as high as possible without strain. Exhale, and lower the right leg. Repeat on the opposite side. This posture can be done prior to the full locust.

Benefits. This posture is a simplified version of the full locust, but the benefits are not as intensive. This posture works on and strengthens the thigh muscles.

Kurmasana — The tortoise

This also activates the manipura chakra.
Sit on the floor with the legs spread as wide as possible. Exhale, and lean forward passing the hands (palms downwards) under the knees. Bring the feet together and cross over the ankles. Slowly bring the head towards the ground, between the knees, and extend the arms behind the buttocks until you are able to clasp them. Hold for as long as is comfortable. On an inhalation, return to the sitting posture.

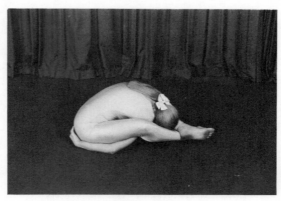

Benefits.   This posture tones the spine and kidneys and removes excess fat from the abdomen. It works on all of the internal organs of the abdomen and helps in ailments such as diabetes, flatulence and constipation. It encourages a fresh flow of blood to the spinal nerves and muscles. It removes headaches, backache and neck pains.

Caution.   Not to be practised by people with slipped discs, sciatica or chronic arthritis.

MEDITATION WITH THE COLOUR ORANGE

Before starting this meditation, read the guidelines which you will find on page 56.

Orange is not often found in conspicuous quantities, and therefore it becomes noticed when it appears amongst other colours. We have to look for it, just as we have to look for joy which is rarely present. This may have to do with the attitudes which we take towards what we have and the gratitude which we should offer every day for these possessions. Gratitude can create joy. Orange, the colour of joy, stands as a small star in the blue of this earth's environment. Blue is often the colour which prompts us to ask questions about our innermost being, of which we usually find only part answers.

When I need to unburden myself from such profound probing, I need this complementary energy, this orange glow of happiness.

So I sit on the grass and behold a marigold which opened this morning to greet the sun. You, little flower, I drink in your colour. You seem to grow. You call me to come and find joy within you. I am seeing myself outside of this happening. I have shut myself out of the communication which can give me joy again. I look at this little flower, the marigold. Am I part of you or are you part of me? How large are you, what size am I? Space and time have changed. I can be within you, right in the middle of this vast, beautiful orange. Joy, linked with deep gratitude, and now, in this no-time existence, I am in joy. I am joy.

I am out of space and time. Space bears no relationship in the space of reality. But what is reality? Is it that which reminds us of the original cause which created. Created this vast marigold. I am like the centre of this flower. It has no size. It is joy, and I am aware of my joy.

Remember then this joy whenever you need to be lifted out of sadness, the heavy moments which cause you to loose heart. Remember that the marigold is there to give you, through gratitude, joy.

Orange marigold, I thank you and I will return to your colour whenever I feel ungrateful and joyless.

THE MANIPURA CHAKRA
OR SOLAR PLEXUS
CENTRE

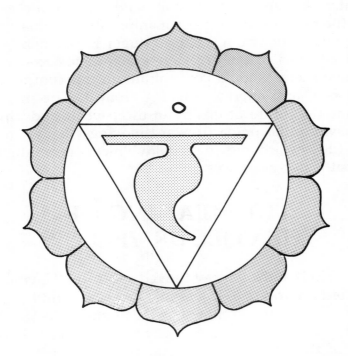

When the senses are stilled, when the mind
is at rest, when the intellect wavers not —
then, say the wise, is reached the highest
stage. This steady control of the senses and
mind has been defined as yoga. He who attains
it is free from delusion.

The Kathopanishad

The word manipura means 'city of jewels'. This chakra is so called because it is the fire centre, the focal point of heat, and is lustrous like a jewel, radiant with vitality and energy. It is depicted as a bright yellow lotus with ten petals. Within the lotus is a red triangle within which sits a ram. The mantra is RAM. The presiding deities are Rudra, consumer or destroyer of the universe, and the goddess Lakini, controller of the flesh element. The solar plexus centre is chiefly concerned with the process of digestion and absorbtion of food. It is said that the adrenal glands, which are located above the kidneys, are a gross manifestation of this chakra. People who suffer from laziness, sluggishness, depression, or malfunctions of the digestive system such as diabetes, indigestion, etc., should concentrate on this centre, trying to feel heat and energy radiating from it. The manipura chakra is the centre of vitality in the psychic and physical bodies where the prana (upward moving vitality) and the apana (downward moving vitality) meet, generating the heat that is necessary to support life.

THE MEANING OF
THE COLOUR YELLOW

Yellow stands at the edge of the red spectrum. Having risen out of red and orange, it loses its heaviness until it finally dissolves into white. Yellow has the energy to detach from gravity and to overcome the physical existence. It is the colour of the ultimate being and it leads into the spirit. When in this state, it points to the future and symbolises in its fine shades the Risen One, He who has overcome all the density of the earth, He who has become an etheric being.

Yellow leads into, and stimulates mental activity. It represents the power of thought and intellect. It can cause envy and abstract remarks which lead into quarrels and arguments. It helps people to detach from obsessional thoughts, feelings and habits.

Yellow light causes a fine change in the biochemical structure. It influences the calcium processes in the physical body and is therefore used in healing for rheumatism and arthritic conditions.

It can reveal that which is not yet complete and shows a person's weaknesses. It can be said that it is the colour to be used in counselling because it can help to release deep-seated problems. When this colour is used for this purpose, the counsellor must be a compassionate person and give protection to the person being counselled.

VISUALISATION ON THE COLOUR YELLOW

For this exercise you will need a piece of yellow material about two metres long and one metre wide. It would be preferable if it were silk and dyed with a natural vegetable dye. If this is not available, a length of yellow cotton material can be used. Before starting this exercise, read about the meaning and qualities of the colour yellow.

Sit down, in a comfortable position, where it is warm and where you will not be disturbed. Take the piece of material and look at it and feel it. Take note of how the material has been woven. Look to see if the colour is uniform throughout or whether it has various subtle shades in it. Gently close your eyes and feel the material. Feel its texture and feel for anything else that it can tell you. Place a piece of the material over the palm of your left hand, then place the palm of your right hand about three centimetres above it. Try to feel the vibrations of the colour. Become aware of whether this colour feels cold, warm or hot. Work with this for about five minutes.

Now take the material and place it around your shoulders. With your eyes closed, try to be aware of any effect that this colour may have on you; whether you feel comfortable or uncomfortable in it; whether any mood changes occur; whether it gives you a feeling of joy or detachment. If you do not like this colour, ask yourself why. Sometimes we will love wearing a colour one day and not be attracted to it the next. When we feel attracted towards a colour, it usually means that there is a quality stimulated by this colour that we need. If you feel opposed to this colour, or any of the other colours, do not stop working with them. Keep trying. You may find that the colours which you dislike will reveal some unknown aspects of your being.

Now sit quietly and try to visualise yellow. During the visualisation take the colour down to the manipura or solar plexus chakra. Feel the colour balancing and energising this centre.

Gently open your eyes and spend a few moments reflecting on anything that you may have experienced. Remove the material from your shoulders and end your visualisation and awareness exercise for today.

MANIPURA YANTRA

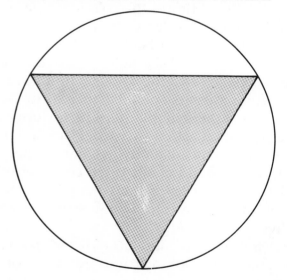

ASANAS WHICH ACTIVATE MANIPURA

Purvottanasana — Intense body stretch

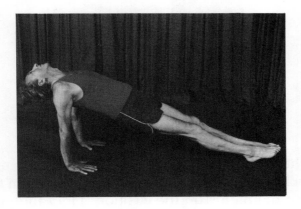

Sit on the floor with the legs stretched out in front. Place the palms of the hands on the floor by the hips, with the fingers pointing in the direction of the feet. Bend the knees, placing the soles of the feet on the floor. Exhale, and lift the body off the floor, taking the pressure on the hands and feet. Keeping the arms straight, straighten the legs and raise the buttocks as high as possible. Take the head back.

Benefits. This posture strengthens the wrists and ankles and works on the shoulder joints. The chest is fully expanded. This asana also helps to relieve minor hip problems.

Ustrasana — The camel

Kneel on the floor with the thighs and feet together. Exhale, placing the right hand on the right heel and the left hand on the left heel. Pressing the feet with the hands and taking the head back, push the spine up until the thighs are in line with the knees. Release the hands, sit back on the legs and

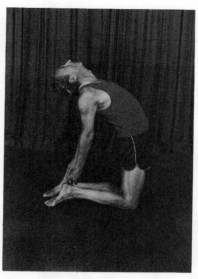

relax. If there is difficulty in keeping the hips in line with the knees, tuck the toes under and place a cushion on the heels. Now place the hands on the cushion. Hold the posture for as long as is comfortable. As you become more supple the posture should be practised without the cushion, and then with the feet lying on the floor without the toes tucked under.

Benefits. This posture stretches and tones the whole of the spine, making it supple. It also works on the abdominal organs and muscles and on the shoulder joints.

Bhujangasana — The cobra

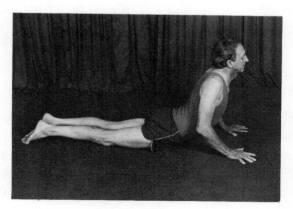

Lie flat on the floor with the chin resting on the floor. Place the hands by the chest with the fingers pointing towards the head. Inhale, and lift the trunk off the floor, keeping the pubis in contact with the floor and the legs straight. Take the shoulders down and back keeping the head in line with the spine. Stay in this posture for as long as is comfortable. Exhale, bend the elbows and come back to the starting position. If your spine is stiff, work with the legs apart, gradually bringing them together as the spine becomes more supple.

Benefits. This posture rejuvenates the spine and is beneficial for stiff backs, lumbago and sciatica. It helps to remove female disorders such as leucorrhea, dysmenorrhea and amenorrhea. It tones the ovaries and uterus. It works on the kidneys and bladder and is good for alleviating water retention. It stimulates the appetite and eliminates constipation.

Caution. Should not be practised by people suffering from an ulcer or hernia.

Dhanurasana — The bow

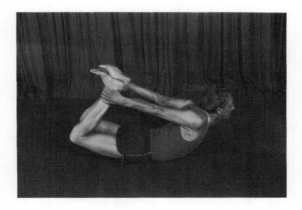

Lie on the floor on the stomach, face downwards. Exhale, bend the knees and hold the ankles with the hands. This is the intermediate position. On the next exhalation, raise the legs and the chest off the floor. Lift the head and take it as far back as possible. Hold this position for as long as is comfortable. Exhale, release the legs and return to the starting position. If you are unable to raise your legs from the floor, work with the intermediate posture until you are able to go into the full posture.

Benefits. This posture stretches the muscles of the abdomen and hips. It tones the muscles of the back and makes the spine flexible. It reduces abdominal fat.

Caution. Not to be practised by people with a hernia or peptic ulcer.

Uttana Mayurasana — The bridge

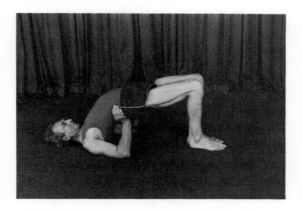

This posture also activates vishuddhi.

Lie flat on the floor. Bend the knees and place the soles of the feet by the buttocks. Inhale, and raise the trunk off the floor, supporting the back with the palms of the hands. Make sure that the hands and elbows are in a straight line. Keep the shoulders on the floor with the neck extended and the knees together. Hold for as long as is comfortable. Exhaling, lower the body back onto the floor. If you have difficulty with this posture, get a wooden block (about the size of a brick) and place it underneath the buttocks. Place the arms on the floor by the side of the raised body. Continue to use your wooden block until you are able to support the body on your hands and arms.

Benefits. This posture strengthens and makes supple the back and wrist joints. It tones the abdominal organs and works on the thigh muscles.

Urdhva Dhanurasana — The wheel

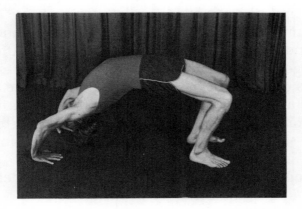

This posture stimulates the remaining six chakras.

Lie flat on the floor, bend the elbows and place the palms of the hands under the shoulders, with the fingers facing towards the feet. Bend the knees and place the soles of the feet by the buttocks. Exhale, and raise the trunk, resting the top of the head on the floor. This is the intermediate posture. On the next exhalation, lift the trunk and head, taking the weight of the body onto the soles of the feet and palms of the hands. Keep lifting up until the arms are straight. Hold for as long as is comfortable. Exhale and lower the body onto the floor. If you are unable to extend into the full posture, work with the intermediate stage until the spine has become supple enough to allow you to go into the full posture.

Benefits.   This posture benefits the entire nervous system and glandular system. It influences all hormonal secretions and relieves various ailments of the female reproductive system. It fully stretches the back, making it supple. It powerfully compresses and massages the abdominal organs.

MEDITATION WITH THE COLOUR YELLOW

Before starting this meditation, read the guidelines which you will find on page 56.

We human beings do not like to be alone and yet we cannot endure the constant company of others. After a time, being together and communicating with a lot of people makes us tired, so we go to sleep. But, is this the only way to withdraw? If the communications have been important and meaningful, if unsolved problems have been brought to mind, to simply withdraw and go to sleep will, in the end, not serve the true growth of consciousness.

To communicate with yourself, you need to detach. The colour yellow is the colour of detachment.

As before, I go onto my path of visualisation. It is the peak of a mountain which I seek. I climb up the mountain, and as I ascend, around me grows a beautiful yellow light. When I reach the summit and stand on the top, I find that I have left all things and people behind me. The yellow shines all around me, I am alone, I am detached. I retreat into my inner self and this yellow of detachment helps me to bring past conversations with my fellow human beings into my soul. It is here that I find the answers to unsolved problems or unanswered questions. I also remember valuable communications which I have had with other people and I build these into my spirit. This enables me to evolve thoughts and ideas, and to share them with others. Standing on this peak of the mountain, I learn to be free. Free from the outer props which keep me in a comfortable social structure that frequently ends up in the meaningless activity of every-day life. Perhaps I would rather not go up onto the peak. However, that will never satisfy me, nor give me the opportunity to bring down from my detached state such gifts of the spirit which I can share, like a beautiful feast, with my fellow people.

Stay in this detached state and ask for the strength and the courage eventually to go back down, but with the knowledge of how to return to this mountain top. Remember that this colour must be approached out of deep trust and with the help of your own higher self. We have to learn again to be alone and silent, but let us make our subsequent journeys to this valuable peak an even greater insight into our true self.

THE ANAHATA CHAKRA OR HEART CENTRE

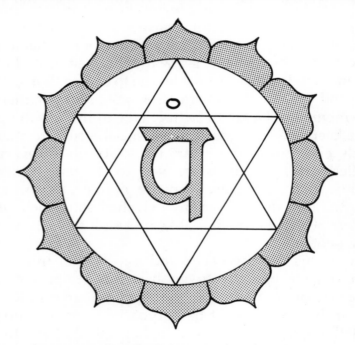

A meditative mind is silent. It is not the silence
which thought can conceive of; it is not the silence
of a still evening; it is the silence when thought — with
all its images, its words and perceptions — has entirely
ceased. This meditative mind is the religious mind — the
religion that is not touched by the church, the temples
or by chants.

The religious mind is the explosion of love. It is
this love that knows no separation. To it, far is
near. It is not the one or the many, but rather that
state of love in which all division ceases. Like beauty,
it is not of the measure of words. From this silence
alone the meditative mind acts.

J. Krishnamurti, Meditations

Anahata means the 'unstruck'. Sound in the manifested universe can be produced by the striking together of objects. This sets up vibrations or sound waves. But the sound which comes from beyond this material world, known as the primordial sound, is the source of all sound. It is the anahata sound. The heart centre is said to be the place where this sound manifests. It may be heard by the yogi as an internal, unborn and undying vibration, the pulse of the universe. The anahata chakra is symbolised by a green lotus with twelve petals. In the centre of the lotus is a hexagram, (as in the Star of David). The mantra is YAM. This is placed on a swift black antelope, the symbol of the Air element. The presiding deities are Isha, the Lord in an all - pervading form, and the goddess Kakini, ruler of the fat element. Anahata is associated on the physical level with the heart and circulatory system, the lungs and respiratory system and the immune system. Sufferers from anaemia, hypertension, palpitations, asthma and bronchitis, should work with this centre.

THE MEANING OF
THE COLOUR GREEN

This is the colour between yellow (rising) and blue (descending). When these two colours enter into a kind of marriage, they cause the colour green to emerge.

Green is the great gift of balance. The colour which offers us the choice to be active or passive. It is the colour which causes materialisation. In green, blue and yellow are always alive. Life has taken hold of matter and is on the brink of death. Out of this most beautiful balance between the Risen One and the descending spirit of renewal, green is the colour of the heart, where we weigh against the feather, according to the Egyptian readings of the Pharaohs. The colour green can also be a strong force to wield.

Considering its healing aspects, green can be used to bring balance into a body which has an over-production of life cells. For example, the illness of cancer. The biochemical reaction on the formation of living cells is to dissolve them before they become permanent.

VISUALISATION ON THE COLOUR GREEN

For this exercise you could use a piece of green malachite. Malachite is one of the oldest known stones and was used a great deal in Egyptian times for its healing properties. It is a stone which absorbs rather than transmits energy. It absorbs negative energy and pain from the human body. Malachite is a balancer of energies, and because of this, it can be used on any of the chakras that are blocked or unbalanced. It is effective when used on the solar plexus. Here it will absorb and release tension, allowing the energy to flow freely again between the upper and lower chakras. If a close relationship with a partner has suddenly ended, this stone can be used on the heart chakra, helping to heal any emotional trauma by absorbing and releasing any pain that this may have caused.

Sit down in a comfortable position, in a place which is warm and where you will not be disturbed. Take the piece of malachite into your hands and observe it. Look at its colour, at its shape and for any patterns that occur in the stone.

Take the stone in your left hand and gently close your eyes. Fold your fingers over the stone, bringing the whole of your concentration into this hand. Try and feel the colour green, the colour of the stone. Feel for any warmth or coldness that this colour emits. Feel the shape of the stone, and any irregularities which occur in that shape. Now ask the stone to tell you of its origin and what properties it has. Sit quietly and listen, keeping your mind concentrated on the stone. Sometimes the stone imparts information to you by the formation of pictures in the mind, at other times by the formation of ideas. Work with this for about ten minutes.

Now take the stone and place it in front of the heart chakra. Feel for the release of any energies from this centre. Visualise the colour being absorbed into this chakra and then radiating out into the aura, bringing about a balance between the negative and positive energies in the body.

When you next practise this awareness exercise, place the stone by the solar plexus chakra. Take note of any differences that you may experience between this and the heart chakra.

Before ending this exercise, spend a few minutes on reflection.

It is important to cleanse this stone after using it (see p. 62).

Another exercise which can be done with this colour, if you have a garden, and weather permitting, is to go out into the garden and stand bare footed on the grass. Close your eyes and direct your awareness to the soles of your feet. Slowly walk around on the grass. Feel the texture and the varying degrees in temperature of the grass through the soles of your feet. Try and discover if the sole of one foot is more sensitive than the other or if you are feeling equally with both soles. Next, try and visualise the green colour of the grass rising up through the soles of your feet into each of the chakras and out into your aura. Feel this colour cleansing the body of all impurities and toxins. Visualise the chakras being cleared of any blockages. Feel the negative and positive energies in the body being balanced. Practise this for about fifteen minutes. Now stand still and notice any changes which may have occurred within you. Gently open your eyes at the end of the exercise.

ANAHATA YANTRA

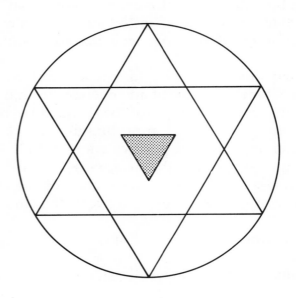

ASANAS WHICH ACTIVATE ANAHATA

Matsyasana — The fish

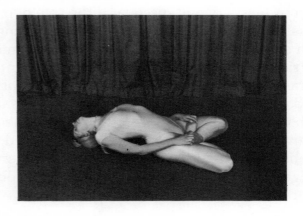

This posture also activates manipura chakra.

Sit in the full lotus posture (see p. 54). Inhale, and on the next exhalation, take the trunk of the body back, supporting it with the arms, until the top of the head rests on the floor. Remove the arms from the floor, and hold the big toe of the right foot with the left hand, and the big toe of the left foot with the right hand. Rest the elbows on the floor, arching the back as much as possible. Hold this posture for as long as is comfortable. Inhale and return to sitting posture.

Benefits. This posture works on the thyroid and parathyroids. The chest is opened up and fully expanded, encouraging deep breathing. It therefore benefits those suffering from asthma or bronchitis. It stretches and tones the abdominal muscles and helps relieve constipation.

Variation 1. For people who are as yet unable to sit in full lotus, lie on the ground, with the legs stretched out. Placing the hands on the ground, arch the back and lower the head onto the floor.

Variation 2. Follow the instruction for Variation 1, but instead of keeping the legs stretched out, bend the right knee and either place the sole of the foot against the inner thigh, or bring the foot onto the thigh as in the half lotus, Repeat with the left leg.

Simhasana

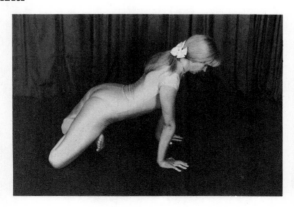

This posture can be practised as a preliminary to Gupta Padmasana (see below).

Sit in full lotus posture. Place the hands onto the floor, in front of the knees, with the fingers pointing forwards. On an inhalation, raise the body onto the knees, pushing the abdomen towards the floor. Hold for as long as is comfortable.

Benefits. This posture works on the organs of the abdomen, especially the liver. It also helps people who have problems with, or who have damaged the coccyx.

Gupta Padmasana — The hidden lotus

Sit in full lotus posture (see p. 54). Place the hands onto the floor, and on inhalation, raise the body onto the knees. Exhaling, slowly lower the front of the body until the chin is resting on the floor. Place the hands behind the back, palms together as in the prayer position. Hold for as long as is comfortable.

Benefits. This posture works on the spine, correcting any postural defects. It opens out and expands the chest cavity and works on the abdominal organs.

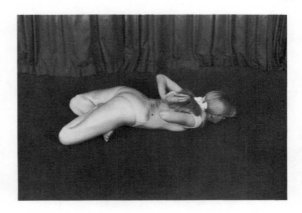

Virabhadrasana 1

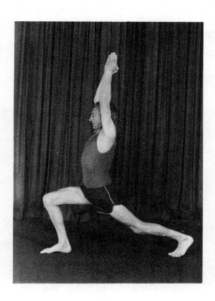

Stand in an upright position, with the feet together, spine straight and shoulders taken back. Inhale, and jump the feet about one metre apart. (People suffering with back problems should 'walk' their feet apart.) Inhale, and turn both of the feet to the right, making sure that the pelvic girdle is in line. Bend the right knee until it is in line with the ankle and forms a 90-degree angle. Keep the back leg straight and lock the knee. On the next inhalation, stretch both of the arms up, until they are straight, and join the palms of the hands over the head. Take the head back. Keep the whole of the concentration on the body, making sure that a right angle is kept with the right knee. Hold for about twenty seconds. Exhale, and come back to standing posture. Repeat on the left side.

Benefits. This posture removes stiffness in the shoulders and back. It fully expands the chest, allowing for deep breathing. It strengthens the ankles and knees, and reduces fat around the abdomen.

Caution. This posture is strenuous and should not be attempted by people with a weak heart.

Virabhadrasana 2

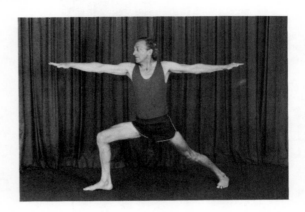

Stand in an upright position with the feet together, spine straight and the shoulders taken back. Inhale, and jump the feet about one metre apart. (People suffering with back problems should 'walk' their feet apart.) Turn the right foot outwards to 90 degrees, and the left foot slightly in to the right. Exhale and bend the right knee to form a right angle, making sure that the knee is kept in line with the ankle. Stretch out the arms horizontally. Turn the head to look at the right hand. Feel as though somebody is holding each of your hands and pulling. Feel the chest being opened and expanded. Hold for about 30 seconds. Inhale, and return to standing posture. Repeat on the other side.

Benefits. This posture opens and expands the chest, allowing for deeper breathing. It strengthens the leg muscles and relieves cramp in the calf and thigh muscles. This posture also helps to strengthen the body.

Baddha Padmasana — Locked lotus

Position 1

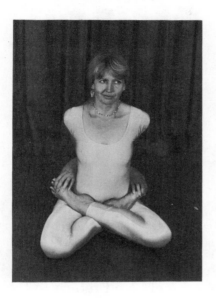

Sit in full lotus posture (see p. 54). Inhale, and clasp the hands behind the back, taking back the shoulders and expanding the chest. On exhalation, slowly bring the body forward until the head touches the floor. Raise the arms and bring them as far as is possible over the head. Hold for as long as is comfortable. On an inhalation, raise the body back to sitting posture. For those who are unable to sit in full lotus, this posture can be practised in half lotus posture.

Position 2

When this posture has been mastered, sit in full lotus and cross the arms over behind the back, attempting to hold the big toe of the right foot with the right hand and the big toe of the left foot with the left hand. Expand and open the

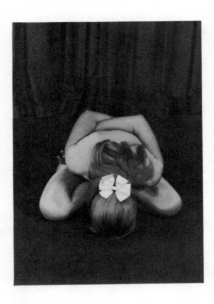

chest as fully as possible. Exhaling, slowly lower the body forward until the head touches the ground. Hold for as long as is comfortable. Inhale, and return to the sitting posture. Release the arms and the legs.

Benefits. This posture alleviates stiffness in the shoulders and arms and expands and opens the chest. It compresses the abdominal organs and thereby helps people suffering from constipation.

Parivrtta Trikonasana — Revolving triangle posture

Stand in an upright position with feet together, spine straight and shoulders back. Inhale, and jump the feet about

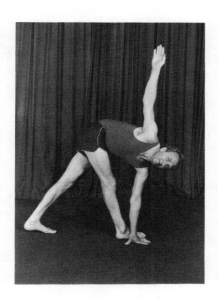

one metre apart. (People suffering with back problems, should 'walk' their feet apart.) Turn both of the feet 90 degrees to the left so that the body is facing to the left with the feet and hips in line. Inhale, and start to rotate the trunk towards the left leg. Exhaling, continue to rotate the trunk, taking the right hand over the left leg, and onto the floor. Stretch the left arm up until it is in line with the right arm, thus fully expanding the chest. Keep both knees locked. Look up at the right hand. Hold for as long as is comfortable. On an inhalation, come back to the standing posture. Repeat on the opposite side. (If you are unable to touch the floor, place a wooden brick or pile of books by the outside of the left foot and place your hand onto these. Aim to make the body supple enough so that the books are no longer needed.)

Benefits. This posture works on the hamstring muscles and thighs. It fully expands the chest and aids in concentration and balance. It invigorates the abdominal organs and strengthens the hip muscles.

MEDITATION WITH THE COLOUR GREEN

Before starting this meditation, read the guidelines which you will find on page 56.

Green is represented by the pivot on a pair of scales. On the right of the scales are all the red colours and on the left all the blue colours. A good balance and equilibrium between two polarities is the green energy. It is the energy which we encounter in plants and trees. Green is a colour which does not take sides.

I need to stand in a neutral place where I can look to either side of this spectrum, and of life. This is the place of those who counsel. I devote all my being to being able to see the truth and in realising that all things have equal importance.

I stand on the green circle. I look to the centre where the green fades into yellow, then into orange and shows me a red centre point.

From this ring of green, I turn my gaze outward. I now see a larger ring of blue which echos some of the green. Then there is a ring of indigo blue. I now see in my mind's eye the archetypal mother energy. Further out is another ring of the purest violet. This whole spectrum of harmonious colour is set into pure white light which has the gentle hue of the peach blossom (magenta).

So I return to my green centre and find my own inner counsellor to balance out my life.

MEDITATION FROM THE HEART CHAKRA

Before starting this meditation, read the guidelines which you will find on page 56.

Find a place which is warm and quiet and where you will not be disturbed. Sit down in a comfortable position, making sure that your spine is straight.

Concentrate on your physical body, trying to release any tension in it. First relax your head, then your neck, your shoulders, your arms and hands, your chest, abdomen, legs and feet. As you release tension, visualise it as a grey mist, floating out of the body and dispersing into the atmosphere. If any part of you feels uncomfortable, change your position to a more comfortable one.

Having relaxed your body, try to relax your mind. Let your mind rest in your breathing and as you breathe out, breathe out any thoughts that come into your mind. If you find that you become lost in these thoughts, gently bring the mind back to the inhalation and exhalation of the breath.

From this concentration on your breathing, move your awareness to your heart. Try to visualise your heart and feel its function. Listen to its slow rhythmic beat. Realise what a marvellous organ the heart is. Moving slightly to the right of your heart, you will find the heart or anahata chakra. Start to walk into this centre. As you enter, you find yourself engulfed in a shaft of pale pink light, the colour of spiritual love. Looking, you see that this light radiates out into the far reaches of the universe, and you feel yourself being gently carried along with it. It takes you out of the room where you are sitting, across your town or county, across the country, the continent, and out into the universe. Glancing back, you see the planet earth bathed in an orb of blue light. As the earth becomes smaller and finally disappears, you discover that you have arrived in a valley filled with pale magenta light.

Standing still, look around at the trees, plants and flowers which are growing here. Some of these display colours that you have not seen on the earth. It is therefore difficult to describe them in words. There are animals running around, playing with each other, completely devoid of fear. Scattered around are stones of all shapes and sizes. Some of these contain colours of variegated design. Bend down and pick up one of these stones. Feel its warmth penetrating your hands. Gazing at it, you are able to see more clearly how the various colours interlace with each other to form the intricate patterns in the stone.

Looking ahead, in the distance, you notice a round white building that looks like a temple. Slowly start to walk towards it. The whiteness of this building looks and feels radiant in the pale magenta light. On approaching this temple, you see a door in front of you. Going up to the door, you push it open and walk inside.

You find yourself in a large circular room filled with white light. Looking round, what catches your attention is a fountain playing in the middle of the room. Walking up to it, you stand and look. It appears different when you compare it with other fountains that you have seen. Considering the amount of water that is cascading down, it is noiseless. Stretch out your arm and place your hand into the water. Immediately your hand comes into contact with the water, you feel all the tension being removed. Your hand becomes heavy and very relaxed. Removing your hand from the water, walk into the middle of the fountain, allowing your body to come into contact with the water.

As you stand there, you feel tiredness, tension and pain being washed away. Your body becomes very relaxed and filled with a surge of energy and joy. You feel as though your old apparel has been washed away and replaced by new. Looking up through the cascading water, you notice a large round window, above the fountain, in the roof of the building. Through this window pours a stream of pure white light. As this light reflects upon the water, it makes each droplet glisten with the different colours of the spectrum. Red, orange, yellow, green, turquoise, blue, indigo, violet and magenta. It makes each droplet have the appearance of a tiny water gem. Ask yourself which colour your body is most in need of. Then, stretching up your arms, catch this coloured water gem in your hands. Feel through the palms of your hands what this colour gem that you have chosen is telling you. Now take it and hold it against any part of your body or by any of the chakras. Place it wherever you feel that it will be beneficial. Feel the colour being absorbed into the body or chakra. Visualise it dispersing any imbalance which may be there. When you feel that it has restored harmony, release it back into the flow of the water. Step out of the fountain and give thanks for what you have experienced.

As you step out, let your gaze wander around the rest of the temple. In front of you, you notice an opening through which comes a golden light. Walk towards the opening and go through. Once inside, you discover that you have entered a small ante-chamber. At first it is difficult to see clearly because of the brilliance of the light. As your eyes become accustomed to the light, you become aware of a being sitting in the room. This being is dressed in white and an emanation of peace and tranquillity flows from it. It bids you to be seated and then invites you to ask any questions that you are seeking an answer to.

These questions could be related to any path that you may be following, problems that you are experiencing, or you may have reached a crossroad in your life and are not sure which way you should take. Ask these things in silence and then sit quietly and listen. The answer may or may not be given immediately. Sometimes answers come through another person, through a book that you pick up to read or from a flash of intuition. But, be assured, that when the time is right, the answer will come. After a few minutes of silence, get up and bid farewell to this being. As you look into its eyes, you experience pure love flowing into you. Turning, you walk out of the ante-room into the main part of the temple. Stand and take one last look at the cascading water of the fountain. With this memory imprinted on your mind, walk to the door of the temple, through the door and out into the valley.

As you walk back along the valley, reflect upon your experiences and feelings.

At the end of the valley, you find the shaft of pale pink light which brought you to this place. Allow it to gently lift you and bring you back to earth consciousness. Travelling down this shaft of light, you enter the earth's atmosphere. You travel over the continent, across the country, across the county or town where you live and back into the room where you are sitting. Be aware of your body sitting on the chair or floor. Visualise a circle of light, which contains a cross of light, and place this around all of your chakras to close them. Start with the crown chakra. Come down to the brow chakra, the heart chakra, solar plexus chakra, sacral chakra and finally the base chakra. As you close the base chakra, feel yourself completely grounded and returned to earth consciousness. Start to increase the inhalation and exhalations of the breath. Now open your eyes and be completely returned.

THE VISHUDDA CHAKRA OR THROAT CENTRE

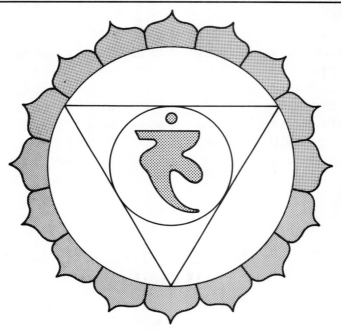

There is a bridge between time and eternity;
and this bridge is Atman, the spirit of man.
Neither day nor night cross that bridge, nor
old age, nor death nor sorrow.

Evil or sin cannot cross that bridge, because
the world of the spirit is pure. This is why
when this bridge has been crossed, the eyes
of the blind can see, the wounds of the wounded
are healed, and the sick man becomes whole
from his sickness.

To one who goes over that bridge, the night
becomes like unto day; because in the worlds
of the Spirit there is a Light which is
everlasting.

from the *Chandogya Upanishad*

The word vishuddha means 'to purify', hence this chakra is the centre of purification. It is symbolised by a smoky violet–blue lotus with sixteen petals. In the centre of the lotus is a white circle. The mantra is HAM. The animal depicted in the chakra is a white elephant which is symbolic of ether. The presiding deity is Ardhanariswara, the form of Lord Shiva and his consort Parvati combined in one body, half male and half female. The goddess of this centre is Sakini, who presides over the element of bone. This chakra influences the vocal chords, the larynx, thyroid and para-thyroid glands. The throat centre is said to be the place where divine nectar or amrita (the mystical elixir of immortality) is tasted. This nectar is a kind of sweet secretion produced by the gland known as the lalana chakra which is located near the back of the throat. By higher yogic practices, the nectar gland is stimulated. The nectar is said to sustain a yogi for any length of time without food or water.

THE MEANING OF
THE COLOUR BLUE

This is the colour which stretches out into space, until ultimately time stands still. The deeper this blue becomes, the deeper is the depth of stillness: the moment of complete arrest is at hand. It is at this point that the blue starts to change into the next colour.

Blue is the colour of peace and of love: the colour of the teacher. It is the colour of infinity, which leads to a new land. Because it creates an experience of space, it is said to be a cold colour. The actual temperature, however, is not influenced by the colour itself. It is the colour which surrounds the earth. It is the sacred blue of the mantel of protection of the Virgin Mary. It is the colour to go into relaxation with and to sleep.

Blue is the colour which surrounds all nature and is the energy of protection. It is also the cradle which will lead into sleep. Those who use the true blue for healing, must be pure in their intentions. This is because they could lead the one who is being healed into such a deep state of relaxation, that ultimately they loose consciousness. If the person needs to be brought into this depth of relaxation and sleep, then he or she must be properly protected.

To use blue for negative purposes, is perhaps the most difficult thing to do. But, if with evil intent, it is achieved, it will render the person who has been put into a state of deep relaxation or sleep, completely vulnerable to the commands and suggestions of another person.

The blue gate is the point through which a soul steps into a new world. As we enter into the New Age, this step should be taken in full consciousness and not in a sleep state. This gate is one of those through which we pass on our way to the ultimate reality. This is represented by the pure white light in which is found all the colours. Blue leads to the spirit and reveals to us our purpose. This comes to pass when we have control over the energy of passion, which is expressed through red, and when this can be transmuted into peace, calm and protection by selfless service to all those whom we meet.

VISUALISATION ON THE COLOUR BLUE

For this visualisation and awareness exercise, you will need a blue flower: a bluebell, iris, cornflower, or any flower that you are able to obtain that has blue petals.

Find a place where it is warm and quiet and where you will not be disturbed. Sit down in a comfortable position. Place the flower in a vase of water in front of you. Close

103

your eyes and try to quieten your mind. Visualise any thoughts coming into the mind as bubbles which float up into the air and gently disperse. Now bring your concentration into the inhalation and exhalation of your breath. With each exhalation, breathe out any tension in the physical body.

When you feel calm and relaxed, open your eyes and take the flower into your hands. Look at each of the petals, Notice how delicate they are. Look for variations in the shapes that the petals form. Notice how they are attached to the stem of the flower. See how many other things you can observe about the formation of this flower. Now be aware of its colour. Are the petals different shades of blue? If so, is the colour lighter at the edges of the petals or near to the stem?

Having absorbed as much information about the flower as you can by observing it, place it on the palm of your left hand, holding the palm of your right hand a few centimetres above it. Close your eyes and try to feel the colour blue. Be conscious of any sensations that you receive through the palm of your right hand. Still with your eyes closed, gently feel the petals of the flower. Compare what you feel with what you observed. When you feel that you have obtained all the information that you are able to, open your eyes and place the flower back into the vase.

Sit for about five minutes and look at the flower. Look at the colour of the petals and try to absorb the colour blue. Now close your eyes and try to visualise the colour blue. As you start to visualise this colour, let the colour grow until it completely surrounds you in an orb of blue light. Feel this orb of light bringing relaxation, peace and tranquillity to the whole of your being. Work with this for five to ten minutes.

At the end of this time, open your eyes and reflect on your experiences before ending the exercise.

VISHUDDA YANTRA

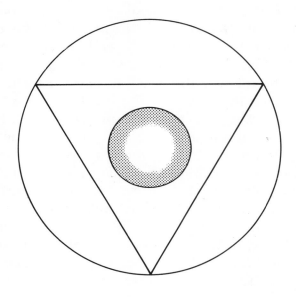

ASANAS WHICH ACTIVATE VISHUDDHA

Halasana — The plough

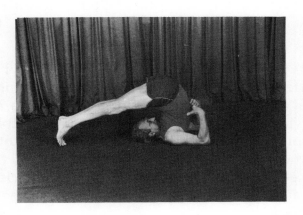

This also activates anahata chakra.

Lie flat on the floor with the arms by the side of the body, palms facing downwards. Make sure that the neck is extended with the chin tucked in towards the chest. On the next exhalation, keeping the legs straight, raise them to 90 degrees. If difficulty is experienced in doing this, bend the knees and then raise the legs. Inhale, and on the next exhalation, take the legs over the head until the feet, with the toes bent under, touch the ground behind the head. Lift up the spine until it is straight. Make sure that the arms are parallel and in line with the shoulders and support the spine with the hands. The chin should be tucked into the chest, forming the chin lock. Hold for as long as is comfortable. Gently roll back onto the floor and relax for a few minutes. People, who, in the beginning, experience difficulty with this posture owing to a stiff back, can place a chair behind the head and lower the feet onto the chair. Keep the legs straight and support the spine with the hands. If difficulty is experienced in keeping the arms parallel whilst supporting the spine, place a belt around the arms, above the elbows, to help you.

Benefits. This posture helps to make supple the spine and back muscles, and therefore benefits the nerves of the spine. It regulates the thyroid gland and balances the metabolic rate. It tones the organs of the abdomen, especially the kidneys, liver and pancreas, thus helping diabetics. It helps to relieve constipation and removes excess fat from the waist.

Caution. This posture should not be practised by the infirm, sufferers of sciatica, back ailments, or high blood pressure. People who have a stiff neck, or who have suffered cervical spine injuries, should practise with blankets. Fold the blankets and place them on top of each other until the right height is found. Place the shoulders and back onto the blankets, allowing the neck and head to be clear of the blankets and to rest on the floor. Now go into the posture.

This allows the neck to be free, thus eliminating any strain. This posture and all inverted postures should not be practised during menstruation.

Sarvangasana — Shoulder balance

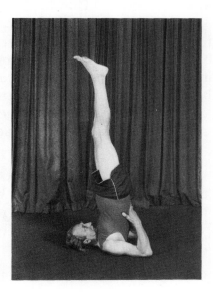

Go into halasana (the previous posture on pages 105–6), Then on an inhalation, raise the straight legs above the head until the body is in a straight line from the shoulders to the toes. With the arms parallel and in line with the shoulders, support the back with the hands. It is important that the neck is extended and the chin tucked into the chest to form the chin lock. There should be no strain on the cervical spine. If the spine or back is stiff, or there has been some injury to the cervical spine, use a blanket as described in the previous posture. The spine should be completely straight and the balance should be on the shoulders and not on the dorsal spine.

Benefits. This posture is frequently known as the mother of postures because it brings harmony into the physical body. The secretions from the thyroid gland have a direct bearing on the reproductive system and also on the hormone secretions from some of the other endocrine glands. Because of the firm chin lock in this posture, the blood supply to the thyroid is increased, thereby helping to regulate the function of this gland. Due to the inversion of the body, more blood is allowed to circulate around the neck and chest, thereby giving relief to sufferers of bronchitis, asthma and throat problems. Also sufferers from prolapse of the bladder and uterus can find relief. Headaches, catarrh and colds can be eradicated with regular practice. It helps menstrual problems, insomnia, hypertension, urinary disorders, hernia and piles. With regular practice a new life and vitality will be felt.

Caution. This posture should not be practised by people with an enlarged liver or spleen or high blood pressure. Even though this posture is beneficial for menstrual problems, it should not be practised during menstruation.

Padma Sarvangasana — Shoulder stand in full lotus

This is the more advanced posture of sarvangasana. Sit on the floor in full lotus (see p. 54). Lean backwards and lie on the floor, with the hands by the sides, palms facing downwards. Exhaling, press down with the hands and raise the folded legs up into the shoulder stand. Support the back with the hands. If necessary, use blankets for this posture as described on page 106. Hold for as long as is comfortable. On the next exhalation, lower the body to the floor, unfold the legs and relax.

Benefits. This posture has the same benefits as sarvangasana, except that the blood from the legs is unable to drain downwards, but the thigh muscles are toned.

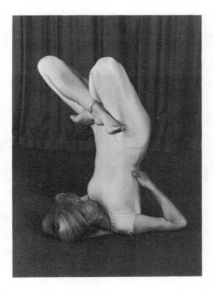

Ardha Chandrasana — The crescent moon

Kneel on the floor with the legs together and arms by the sides. Bring the sole of the right foot onto the floor, making a right angle with the knee. On an inhalation, stretch the left leg backwards and place the hands, palms downwards, on either side of the right foot. Exhale. On the next inhalation, continue to move the leg backwards, whilst arching the back and taking the head back. Allow the hands to come off the floor until just the fingertips are touching. Exhale, and return to kneeling position. Repeat on the other side.

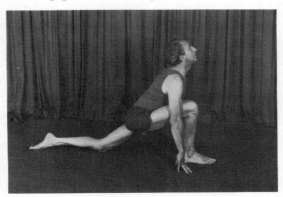

Benefits.   This posture strengthens and makes supple the whole of the skeletal structure.

Variation.   For increased benefits, raise the arms over the head, stretching the head and upper trunk as far back as possible.

MEDITATION WITH THE COLOUR BLUE

Before starting this meditation, read the guidelines which you will find on page 56.

In times of activity, there is always the speed and the rush which allows us no rest and no peace. I am driven. I must be active. The peaceful times of relaxation, when I can just be, fade into the background and become an unobtainable dream.

I close myself into an orb of blue light which takes the shape of a cradle or hammock. All the things around me becomes circular and veiled in blue. Time slows down. I am no longer being driven. I am completely relaxed, but in no way passive. I experience the energy of blue and the unobtainable dream is now reality. I am peace, I am completely relaxed. I realise that I can be the master of this absolute peace. I am in the arms and on the lap of this timeless mother being, the queen of the kingdom where peace and protection are one and the same energy. I can now create a time which feels like eternity when in the physical reality; only a fraction of a second has passed. I stay in this blue orb and learn through it, that I can create its peace and relaxation by using the image of blue.

I now return to the room where I am sitting but now know that I am able to create this state of peace and relaxation using the colour blue, at any time. Also, if I wish, I can extend this peace and love to all of the friends that I meet on life's journey.

THE AJNA CHAKRA OR THIRD-EYE CENTRE

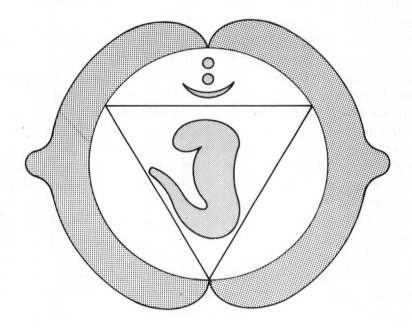

The sound of Brahman is OM. At the end of
OM there is silence. It is a silence of joy.
It is the end of the journey where fear and
sorrow are no more: steady, motionless, never-
falling, ever-lasting, immortal. It is called
the omnipresent Vishnu.

In order to reach the highest, consider in
adoration the sound and the silence of Brahman.
For it has been said:

God is sound and silence. His name is OM.
Attain therefore contemplation — contemplation
in silence on him.

From the *Maitri Upanishad*

This chakra is sometimes known as the brow or third eye. The word ajna means 'command'. Through this chakra one is able to obtain a deeper level of meditation and to come into contact with the higher self. It is depicted as a two-petalled lotus manifesting a deep, indigo, violet colour. The two petals represent the positive and negative aspects of prana, which meet at this centre through the ida and pingala nadis. The mantra is 'AUM', and the presiding deities are Paramshiva, the formless consciousness and the goddess, Hakini, who controls the subtle mind. Of all the centres, this is the one best known and most used by people of all paths and disciplines for concentration and meditation. The point which is usually concentrated on is between the eyebrows, but the place where the centre is situated is within the area of the brain. In the physical body it is related to the pineal and pituitary glands. The pineal gland is about the size of a pea and is almost atrophied in adulthood. On the psychic level, it is said to be the bridge between the physical, mental and psychic bodies. When this chakra is awakened, one is given the gifts of clairvoyance, clairaudience, telepathy and other psychic gifts, which in most people lie dormant. Through sensitivity, it is possible to transmit and pick up thought energy through ajna. Likewise, one can send colour through this centre to a person who has asked for absent healing. On a physical level, when this centre is stimulated, it can heighten intelligence, memory, willpower and concentration.

THE MEANING OF
THE COLOUR INDIGO

The blue deepens and leads into the vast spaces of the heavens, where in the deep, deep silence of these spaces a new life movement appears. Because of the depth of this colour, it is difficult to see with the outer eye. We must therefore open the inner eye and experience images of life before they become manifest on the physical plane. If we are in a darkened room, lit by just a candle, and we close our eyes, the colour of indigo will arise in that vast expanse which is within us. Images then start to appear. They 'dance' and move. They evolve and dissolve. When we become still enough, this indigo colour will show us the inner world of the spirit, in order to prepare us for that light which appears when we learn to let go, live in the now and just be.

Indigo represents the curtain which veils us from the light of the true spirit. When we are ready, this curtain is gently dissolved, revealing the light of the spirit and the purpose behind creation. To achieve this state, we must let go of the material world and ask to be shown the origins of this unmanifested world. It is in this deep indigo where the images gently appear, that we are persuaded to look and not forced to see.

VISUALISATION ON THE COLOUR INDIGO

For this exercise, you will need a sheet of paper, a paintbrush, some indigo and white paint and a coloured picture of the ajna yantra. Take these things to a quiet and warm place where you will not be disturbed.

Sit down and look at the yantra. Look at its shape and colours. Notice how the deep indigo becomes lighter as it moves towards the centre of the circle, and then, having reached the centre, becomes pure white. As you observe this yantra, try to interpret what it symbolises for you.

Now take your paint and paintbrush and try to copy it onto your piece of paper. It does not have to be exact or perfect. As you paint, be aware of your feelings for this colour. Do you like it? Does it recall any past incidences in your life? If you like the colour, can you visualise how you would like to use it, either in your home or upon yourself? If you don't like the colour, ask yourself why not. As you move towards the lighter shades at the centre, do your feelings change?

When you have finished the painting, place it on the palm of your left hand and hold the palm of your right hand above it. Close your eyes and try to feel the vibrations through the palm of your right hand. If you practise this regularly, you should be able to feel several different vibrations, that of indigo, the light blue and the white. When you first practise with this colour, you may not feel anything. Do not be disappointed and give up. Stay with this awareness for about five minutes.

Now, with your eyes still closed, take an imaginary paint brush and paints, and imagine that you are painting the yantra in the space in front of your eyes. Visualise the colour as your imaginary picture grows. When you have completed it, place it in front of the ajna chakra. Feel the white at the centre radiating out and clearing any blockages that may be present.

After a little while, replace the white with the indigo and watch as this colour brings the energies of the ajna chakra into balance. Gently open your eyes and reflect upon your experiences with this exercise before you end your session for the day.

When you next work with this exercise, do not use the painting that you have just created, but make a new one. The act of painting with colour helps one to visualise and become sensitive to it.

AJNA YANTRA

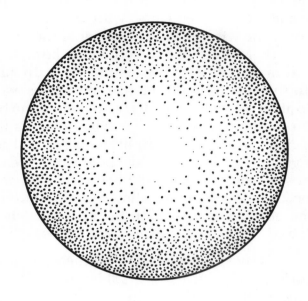

ASANAS WHICH ACTIVATE AJNA

Gomukhasana — The cowhead

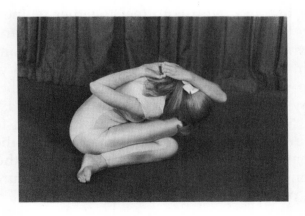

Sit on the floor with the legs stretched out in front. Bend the left knee and take the left foot under the right leg placing the heel of the foot by the right buttock. The knee should be on the floor making a straight line with the hip. Taking the right leg over the left leg, place the heel of the right foot by the left buttock. Make sure that both knees lie on top of each other. If, through stiffness, you are unable to do this, gently work with the posture until the legs and knees assume the correct position. Now take the left arm behind the back with the hand reaching up as far as possible towards the head. Take the right arm over the right shoulder and join both hands. If you are unable to do this, hold a belt in each hand, slowly moving the hands up the belt until they meet. The arm going over the shoulder should be in a straight line, behind the head. Inhale, and on the next inhalation, bring the trunk and head down towards the knees.

Benefits. This posture alleviates stiffness in the knees, thigh muscles, neck, arms and shoulder joints. It also opens up the chest. It stimulates the kidneys and pancreas, thereby helping sufferers of diabetes. Tension is relieved in the spine and back muscles. It also helps to relieve sciatica and rheumatism.

Nataraja Asana — Lord Shiva's posture

Stand on the floor with both feet together, spine straight, shoulders back and chest open. Fix your gaze on an object in front of you and feel your body in a state of balance. Bend your right knee, and taking the right leg behind you, hold the ankle with the right hand. Inhaling, raise the leg and foot away from the body whilst raising them as high as possible. Now extend the left arm upwards and forwards, fixing your gaze on the left hand. Make sure that the knee of the leg that you are balancing on is locked. Hold the posture for as long as is comfortable. Exhale and return to the standing posture. Repeat on the opposite side.

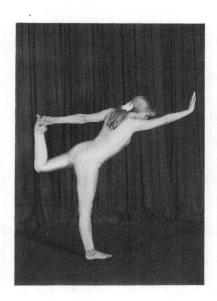

Benefits. This posture develops balance and concentration and makes the legs strong and supple.

Hanumanasana — The splits

Kneel on the floor. Bend the right knee, placing the sole of the foot onto the floor. Place the palms of both hands onto the floor on either side of the body. Gently slide the right leg forwards and the left leg backwards, taking the weight of the body on the arms and hands. Keep extending the legs

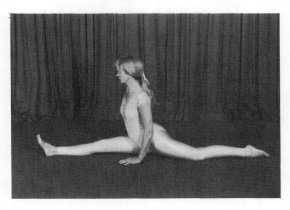

until they are straight and lying on the ground. Keeping the balance, join the palms of the hands in front of the chest. Hold for as long as is comfortable. Come back to the kneeling posture and repeat on the other side. This posture can take a long time to master, but with regular practice and perseverance, it can be obtained.

Benefits. This posture improves the blood circulation in the legs, thighs and hips, and tones the leg muscles. It relaxes and strengthens the abductor muscles of the thighs and helps sufferers of sciatica.

Ardha Matsyendrasana — Half abdominal twist

Sit on the floor with the legs straight out in front. Bend the right knee, taking the right leg over the left leg and placing the sole of the foot on the floor by the left knee. Bend the left knee, placing the heel of the foot by the right buttock. Turn the trunk of the body towards the right, taking the left arm over the right knee, bend the elbow and open the palm of the hand outwards. Place the palm of the right hand on the floor, behind the body, with the fingers pointing away from the body. Keeping both buttocks on the floor and exhaling,

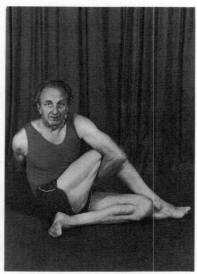

rotate the trunk as far to the right as possible, looking over the right shoulder. Hold for 30 to 60 seconds. On an inhalation, return to the starting position and repeat on the other side.

Benefits. This posture makes the spine and back muscles supple, helping to eliminate lumbago and muscular rheumatism. Because this posture works on the spine, it also works on the spinal nerves. It massages the abdominal organs and removes digestive ailments. It tones the kidneys, adrenal glands and pancreas. It is therefore a good posture for people suffering from diabetes.

MEDITATION WITH
THE COLOUR INDIGO BLUE

Before starting this meditation, read the guidelines which you will find on page 56.

In this day and age, we work mostly with only one half of the brain. If we are not careful, this could chain us to the prison walls of pure logic. In our deep subconscious, most of us are aware of this, but we now lack the courage to use our imaginations which in most people is representative of the right side of the brain, where all the original images of life came from. The old masters call this inner eye the third eye.

I can, with this third eye, make pictures which no camera can produce. I can add to a beautiful human being wings and a halo. I can see that being standing on a moon sickle with stars around its head. In other words I can paint pictures which come from a world in which logic and mathematics have no place. On the negative side, I could also allow my imagination to become an uncontrollable force which makes me lose my bearings here on earth. When I am using my clear consciousness and remain the conductor of this force of inspiration and imagination, then I can start

119

to create healing images which are not based only on the logical medical health patterns, but which have their origin in the vast spaces of superconsciousness.

I use this indigo blue as the cosmic, etheric, rejuvenating energy. These energies, which I had forgotten, start to flow to me. I experience now this flow of life and it contains the messages for my complete life. I let myself be free to accept what I have inadvertently neglected, not realising that it had almost taken away from me that full life of which I can avail myself. Deep in this indigo blue, a touch of violet comes and it shows me, in sparkles of gold, a spiritual reality.

It is very deep and full of the sacred darkness and yet not dark. It contains life everlasting. It is the source of existence and full of the wealth of creation which includes me and all life upon which I depend.

Now I close my eyes. I go into this deep indigo blue. The world around me is not there any more. In my in-breathing, I experience a beautiful tingling sensation which seems to enliven every cell of my body. I see in this wonderful spaceless realm a still night sky, which has no clouds and no stars. As a little time passes, the indigo blue becomes brilliant and shining as if it is an invisible light. Pure deep energy surrounds me and I begin to encounter a mysterious presence. I ask for healing images — there — wait, is it or is it not the most perfect face of a most highly evolved being. Everything about it is so immaculate that I can only sense it to be a risen, completed god image. It now speaks to me.

'Hold in your inner eye this perfection, it is what you asked of me, the complete being. It will heal all that is at present not well. See me in all other human beings and you will be able to heal them also.'

The image fades into this deep glowing indigo, but it leaves behind an invisible energy. I can ask many questions and each one will find an answer. So I now know where to go when I need inspiration. I stay for a while silently in this life-embued space. Thank you. My world is no longer surrounded with limitations. Thank you for the world beyond this world. Thank you for indigo blue. I close my inner eye and prepare to open the outer eyes slowly, thus returning to everyday consciousness as I have been instructed.

THE SAHASRARA CHAKRA OR CROWN CENTRE

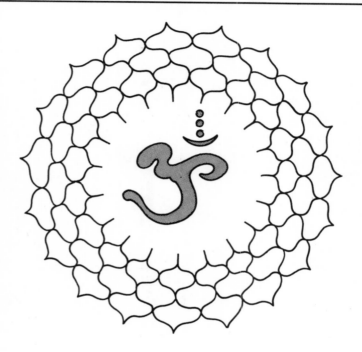

Crown of God, highest aspiration,
fulfilling the plan of all plans.
Eternal consciousness
without beginning.
That always was, that always is
and will never end.
Crown of God, immeasurably beautiful.
God the Father, God the Mother,
God the Daughter, God the Son.
Crown of unity, crown of the absolute.
Woven of light, light of the eternal.
Created out of darkness,
the fountain of all being

contained in the timeless, spaceless existence.
It is
not nothingness.
Nothingness is it.
Silence and the harmony of the spheres,
the one sphere not measured
It is.

Theo. Gimbel

In yoga, the sahasrara centre is not looked upon as a chakra but as the abode of the highest consciousness. It is situated above the head and depicted as a thousand-petalled lotus. A thousand represents eternity, something which has no ending. In the centre of the lotus is a shivalinga, the symbol of pure consciousness. It is said that in this centre the mystical union of Shiva (consciousness) and Shakti (matter and energy) takes place, the individual being with the supreme being. In yogic and tantric philosophy, the universe is said to have manifested by the separation of these two forces. When the dynamic force of kundalini is awakened, it rises through the chakras to the sahasrara centre and merges into the force from whence it came. This must only happen when a person is ready physically, mentally and spiritually and not awakened by force, which can be dangerous. One is then brought into a state of pure consciousness, the ultimate goal of yoga. When this has been attained, the yogi gains supreme knowledge and passes beyond life and death.

THE MEANING OF
THE COLOUR VIOLET

The moment of stillness has passed and we step out of deep indigo. A drop of red love has fallen into this indigo and changed it into violet. Violet, the colour which has now been created leads us into the spiritual worlds. Here dignity

123

rises and brings with it the energy of divinity, the awe, the respect of self, and the one who can acknowledge the kingship of God, and by this enters into the state of the priest. The shining colour of violet lifts the prepared being into this higher state, to be accepted as a priest or priestess. Violet leads us into the realm of the spirit awareness and is the last gateway before the true self is apparent.

In healing, this colour can restrengthen a weak cell structure and rebuild energy where the loss of this is experienced. With this, we are entering into the first spiritual feminine colour.

A negative use is the withholding of this colour from those in need of it. This colour can make a person feel they are too good to do any of the down-to-earth work. With this superior air, they imagine that some of the daily tasks are too dirty and unclean for them to touch. This is pride without the protection of humility.

In the true sense of this colour is brought about the birth of humility. — not the humility which causes a feeling of unworthiness, but humility which brings about humble pride.

The person who is able to accept this colour, transforms the negative side of pride into the positive. When pride becomes veiled in the grace of violet, it leads us to the last gate before the ultimate reality.

VISUALISATION ON THE COLOUR VIOLET

For this exercise in visualisation and awareness, you will need a piece of amethyst.

Amethyst is a powerful healing stone and comes in light and dark shades of violet. The lighter shades can be used for mysticism and spiritual inspiration, whereas the darker shades act as powerful transformers of energy. These darker shades work with the kundalini energy, balancing and stabilising the base chakra. The amethyst is a stone of inspiration and humility, reflecting the love of God. It is a wonderful stone to use in healing, especially in conjunction with colour healing. It helps both physical and emotional pain.

Find a place which is quiet and warm and where you will not be disturbed. Sit down in a comfortable position, either on the floor or on a chair.

Place the piece of amethyst in front of you and look at it carefully. Take note of what form the crystal or crystals take, and how the light is reflected through the stone. Look for any variation in the colour.

Pick up the stone and hold it in your hands, remembering that crystals contain life force. Feel the shape and texture of this crystal. Now close your eyes and feel through your hands for any vibrations that this stone is radiating. Ask the stone to tell you of its origin. Then watch for any pictures or thoughts which come into your mind. Open your eyes and look once more at the colour of the crystal. Closing your eyes, try to visualise this colour of violet. Mentally take this colour into the crown chakra, allowing it to balance and energise this centre. If you are experiencing any emotional pain, take this colour into the heart chakra and hold it there until the pain starts to ease.

When you are ready, open your eyes. Be conscious of anything that you may have experienced during this time. Cleanse your crystal as described on page 62 and put it in a sunny place to be energised in readiness for when you next use it.

SAHASRARA YANTRA

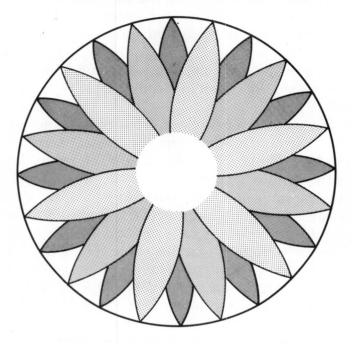

ASANAS WHICH ACTIVATE SAHASRARA

Prasarita Padottanasana — The expanded-foot posture

Stand in an upright position with the feet together, spine straight, shoulders back and chest expanded. Inhale, and jump or walk the feet about 1 metre apart. Make sure that the feet are parallel and the toes in line. Exhaling, and keeping the spine straight, extend the trunk forward from the hips, placing the palms of the hands on the ground, fingers facing forwards. If the body is stiff and the hands cannot reach the floor, use a wooden brick or books to put the hands on. This is the intermediate posture. Now, slowly walk the hands backwards until they are in line with the

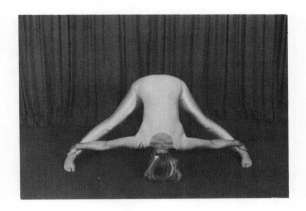

feet, at the same time extending the trunk until the top of the head rests on the floor between the hands. Once this position has been mastered, the hands can be placed behind the back in the prayer position. Alternatively, the left hand can hold the left ankle and the right hand the right ankle. Hold this posture for as long as is comfortable. Inhaling, come back to the intermediate position. Exhale, and on the next inhalation, return to standing posture and bring the feet together.

Benefits. This posture works on the inner thighs and hamstring muscles. It removes stiffness from the shoulders and fully opens the chest. A fresh supply of blood flows to the head, neck and trunk of the body. This posture can be done by people who are unable to do the full head balance.

Bhumi Pada Mastakasana — The half headstand

This is the preliminary pose for the full head balance. Kneel on the floor on all fours. The knees and legs should be about 15 centimetres apart, and the palms of the hands, fingers facing forwards, should be in line with the knees, and with the shoulders. Place the crown of the head on the floor between the hands. Straighten the legs, taking the balance onto the head and feet. Take the hands behind the back into

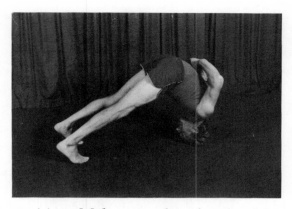

the prayer position. Make sure that the shoulders are taken back in order to fully open the chest. To start with, hold this posture for about 15 seconds, gradually increasing the length of time. Bring the hands back onto the floor, bend the knees and lie down on the floor in relaxation for a few minutes.

Benefits. This posture strengthens the neck and back muscles. It relieves stiffness in the shoulder joints and fully expands the chest. The fresh supply of blood to the head invigorates the brain and face and is good for people with low blood pressure. This posture also works on the hamstring muscles in the legs.

Caution. This posture should not be practised by people with cervical spine problems, high blood pressure or sufferers of vertigo.

Bakasana — The crane

Kneel on the floor on all fours. Make sure that the hands are in front of the knees and in line with the shoulders. Place the crown of the head on the floor about 15 centimetres in front of the hands, thus making a triangle with the head and hands. Walk the feet towards the hands, straightening the spine. Bend the left knee and place on the left arm. Bend the right knee and place on the right arm. Bring the feet

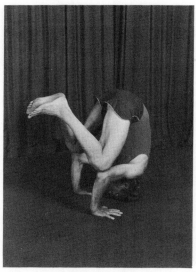

together to form the tail of the bird. Hold for one to two minutes. Bring the legs down and relax.

Benefits. This posture helps one to gain a sense of balance and is also a good preliminary asana to the head balance. It strengthens the arms and wrists and gives a fresh supply of blood to the head, face and neck.

Sirasana — Head balance

Beginners should practise this posture against a wall until balance and confidence have been gained. Fold a blanket and place it on the floor in front of the body. Kneel on the floor in front of the blanket. Clasp your hands, and, bending the elbows, place them on the blanket. Make sure that the lower arms are parallel and the elbows in line with the shoulders. Place the crown of the head onto the blanket between the cupped hands, so that the back of the head touches the palms of the hands. Straighten the legs, bringing the feet onto the floor. Slowly walk the feet towards the head until the thighs come into contact with the abdomen.

129

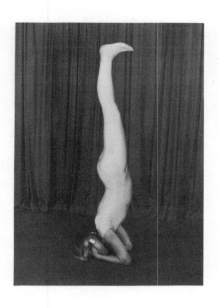

Lift up the spine and gradually take the balance and weight of the body onto the arms and head. Now slowly take the feet off the floor. When your balance feels secure, straighten the legs. Once in the head balance, lift up the body from the shoulders, making sure that there is no pressure on the cervical spine. Make sure that the body is straight. The whole of your concentration should be on the body, making minor adjustments where necessary. When a person first starts to practise sirasana, it should be held for about 30 seconds. With practice, the time is gradually increased until the posture can be held for 30 minutes. When coming out of the head balance, slowly bend the knees and bring the feet back onto the ground. Go down into the pose of a child and relax. If one immediately stands up, the blood which had been circulating in the head and neck, suddenly drains away, leaving one feeling giddy.

This posture can be practised with a chair. Place the chair behind you, and instead of going up into the full head balance, placing the feet onto the chair. Walk the feet forwards on the chair until the spine is straight.

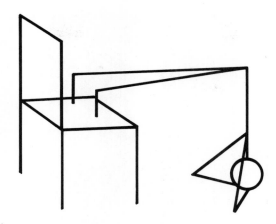

Benefits. Sirasana is known as the king of all postures. It increases the flow of blood to the brain thus rejuvenating the cells and making its function more efficient. It ensures a good blood supply to the pituitary and pineal glands, thus ensuring a greater sense of well being and vitality. Owing to the reverse flow of the blood, it helps tired legs and varicose veins. Through the inversion of the body, prolapses of the bladder and uterus are helped. It relieves headaches and is beneficial for colds and asthma.

Caution. This posture should not be practised by people with high blood pressure, neck problems, heart palpitations, thrombosis, chronic catarrh, chronic constipation, detached retina or glaucoma. It should also not be practised during menstruation.

Salamba Sirasana

Practise this posture against a wall until you have mastered its balance. Kneel on the floor and follow the instructions for bakasana, the crane posture. From bakasana lift the legs up straight until you come into the head balance. To start with hold for about 30 seconds, gradually increasing the time to

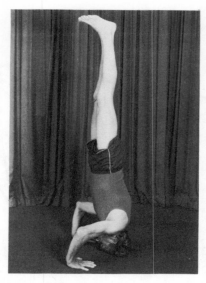

30 minutes. Exhale and bring the legs back to bakasana. Hold for a few seconds. Come back to the kneeling posture, then lie on the floor and relax.

Benefits. This has the same benefits as sirasana with the addition of strengthening the abdominal muscles through raising and lowering the legs from and back into bakasana.

Caution. The same as for sirasana.

MEDITATION WITH
THE COLOUR VIOLET — I

For this meditation, you need to fall back on your memory and imagine that you are standing in your garden or in the open space of a field in the early hours of the morning. Dawn has not yet broken. You are free from all civilisation, alone and in silence.

Lie down and look up into the sky. Looking deep into the universe, it gives an indigo–violet background to the stars which are shining. You watch as it changes into a pure violet colour. This violet colour seems to come down, folding itself around you. All other colours have gone, leaving just this pure violet, filled with the stars which look like golden specks against its background. This is space, the temple of God, the holy silent energy. It says, 'Love yourself, respect yourself, accept dignity and know that you are a microcosm of this universe.' Let go of time and space in this beautiful violet colour and feel at peace with all things around you; the earth, the water, the fire, the air and the life forces which are within you.

Visualise yourself as a perfect spiritual being, knowing that you can be this being if you allow yourself to be. Realise that your fine and valuable thoughts make you a being who can influence the plan of this vast world around you. Welcome the emotions and feelings that you are experiencing at this moment. Look at joy and sorrow, love and hate, comfort and pain as if you are seeing the whole of your soul as part of the universe in which these feelings belong not only to you, but to all things. Look upon this experience as part of your growth pattern.

Be aware that your body is a temple in which is celebrated the transformation of earthly nourishment into the life-force energies. The spiritual energies have let trickle down such unimaginable fine substances in order to allow the life forces to create seeds and plants, fruits and vegetables from which we gain this nourishment. In the violet colour of dignity, the transforming is like a holy communion on a higher level.

Your body, made of flesh, was formed out of the original seeds of your parents. You are now the conductor of this beautiful instrument. You are bathed in this violet light and are worthy to be chosen as priest/priestess of the universe. You are the physical representative of the divine world.

You are lying down, looking up into the sky at night. You have been on a journey from which you must now return. Be aware of being in the open space of a field or in your garden. Come back to it and with thanks accept the new day which is about to break. You cannot return to yesterday, so why not make this the first day of the rest of your life and start this first day in dignity and gratitude for the beauty of your own being.

Take in a deep gentle breath and fill your lungs. Move your limbs carefully, they deserve a loving gentle movement. When you are ready, open your eyes. Carry within you this newly awakened memory of who you really are. You have grown and realised more about yourself during this meditation. Carry this within you with humble pride or proud humility.

MEDITATION WITH THE COLOUR VIOLET — II

How often do I feel unworthy and look down upon myself? I have to some extent still to overcome the shame that my parents and even my grand-parents made me feel when I did not behave in the way that they wanted me to. I am not perfect, and never will be, but I can achieve peaks when I am, for a moment or for a day, feeling that I am a person who is worthy, who has dignity and who treats him/her self with self-respect . . .

The colour violet is the colour of grace. A colour that uplifts my heart, my soul and myself into the higher spirit consciousness.

I have never premeditatively done anything to take away from others. I have not deliberately despised or maljudged my fellow beings. On account of this, I should now forgive myself, my parents and those who may have made me feel undignified. In humble pride, I should see myself as one of the essential souls in the plan of this world.

I wrap around me the cloak of violet and see myself in the temple of reverence. I am at this moment, the only person who can add to the plan, that which is needed for all to attain divinity. Someone did this yesterday, someone will do it tomorrow, but now, today, I am that being. Grace,

134

beauty and divinity I offer in order to serve in this temple which is like a beautiful violet flower.

This is the paramount sensation, my own offering to the universe. I am now made into the priestess or the priest. This is not of my own volition, but it has made me the channel through which can now flow this dignity and respect. I can see all things around me being graceful and I can not imagine them in any other way. They are all lifted up to the condition into which I have now been elevated. Amongst those who I now see are my neighbours, family, friends and people in the place where I live. How can I have missed out on this incredible grace? Thank you Universe. Thank you Spirit. Thank you angelic kingdom.

I now prepare myself, as I have been instructed, to return from this temple of violet to the room where I have been meditating.

BALANCING AND ENERGISING THE CHAKRAS

For this relaxation and awareness exercise you can either sit or lie down in a place where it is warm and where you will not be disturbed. If you choose to lie down, you can cover yourself with a blanket. In this exercise, each inhalation and exhalation of the colours is to the count of five. The visualisation of each of the colours coming into the chakra and radiating out into the aura is repeated five times.

Having made your body comfortable, gently start to quieten your mind. Try to let go of any problems or plans that you are trying to make. Let go of the things that you have been doing or things that you have yet to do. Bring that quietened mind into your breathing. Be aware of the gentle inhalation and exhalation of the breath. With each exhalation feel the body releasing tension and the metabolism slowing down. Feel the slow and regular beat of the heart.

Now bring your concentration down into both of your feet. Feel for any tension in the muscles of the feet and try to let go of this tension. Feel your feet becoming very relaxed and heavy. Move up into your legs. Feel your ankles, your calves and shins, your knees and your thighs. Be aware of the muscles in your legs. Feel for any tension in these muscles and try to let go of it. Let your legs become relaxed and with this relaxation feel them getting heavier. Move your attention up into your abdomen. Visualise the pelvic girdle, the muscles which support and surround this and the organs which are contained within the abdominal cav-

136

ity. Relax. Let go of any tension in this part of the body. Feel your abdomen becoming heavier and heavier. Bring your concentration up into the solar plexus. This is an area where a lot of nervous tension can be felt.

The solar plexus chakra is frequently over active. Feel for any tension here and let go of it. Visualise this tension as a grey mist floating away from the body and dissolving. As this mist floats away, feel your solar plexus becoming very heavy and relaxed. Next move your concentration up into your chest. Visualise the rib cage, the muscles which support and surround this skeletal structure and the organs which are contained within the chest cavity. Feel the slow and rhythmic beat of the heart, remembering that your heart is a large muscular organ. Be aware of the slow inhalation and exhalation of the breath. Know that with each inhalation you are breathing in prana or life force, that which energises and vitalises your whole being and without which you would not be alive.

Feel for any tension in the organs and muscles of the chest. Consciously let go of this tension and feel your chest becoming very, very heavy and relaxed. Now move your concentration up into your neck and head. Relax your throat and all the muscles surrounding your neck. Relax your tongue, your jaws, your cheeks, your eyes, your forehead, the top and the back of your head. Feel your neck and your head becoming heavy with relaxation.

Lastly, bring your concentration into your spine. Feel the spine from the coccyx (the tail bone) up through the sacrum, lumbar, thorasic and cervical vertebrae. Feel the muscles which surround and support the spine. Also be aware that the main nervous system runs through the spine. Feel for any tension in this part of the body. Let go of it so that your spine becomes so heavy that it feels as though it is sinking into the floor. Be aware also that the spine is that instrument which grounds us to this planet earth but through which we are also able to be lifted up into the higher realms of consciousness. Now be aware of your whole physical body.

Be aware of it in a state of complete relaxation, completely free from tension.

With your body in this state of relaxation, bring your concentration into the base or muladhara chakra. On the next inhalation, visualise a beam of pure red light coming through the soles of your feet into this centre. Feel its warmth and feel how it grounds you to this earth. As you exhale, let this colour radiate out into your aura.

Move your concentration up into the swadisthana chakra. Inhaling, visualise a beam of pure orange light coming through the soles of your feet, up through your legs and into this centre. Feel the joy and energy of this colour filling the whole of your being. Exhaling, let it flow out into your aura.

Bring your concentration up into the manipura or solar plexus chakra. On the next inhalation, visualise a beam of pure yellow light coming through the soles of your feet, up into this centre. Feel this colour releasing any tension or blockages in this part of the body. Exhaling, watch the colour radiating out into your aura.

Next bring your concentration up into the anahata or heart chakra. Inhaling, visualise a beam of pure green light horizontally entering this chakra. Feel it balancing this centre and balancing both the negative and positive energies in the body. Exhaling, watch it as it flows out into your aura.

Shift your concentration up into the vishuddha or throat chakra. Inhaling, bring a beam of clear blue light through the top of your head into this centre. Feel the peace and tranquility that this colour brings with it. Allow it to release any tension that you may have found difficult to release. Exhaling, allow the colour to flow out into your aura.

Bring your concentration up into the ajna or brow chakra. Inhaling, bring a beam of pure clear indigo light through the top of your head into this centre. Allow this colour to give you a clearer insight into any path which you may be following and the work which you have chosen to do in this

138

lifetime. Exhaling, allow it to radiate out into your aura.

Finally, bring your concentration up into the sahasrara or crown chakra. This is situated just above the top of the head. Inhaling, visualise a beam of pure clear violet light entering this centre. Feel this colour giving you the dignity that you should have as a human being. Exhaling, allow it to radiate out into the aura. As it radiates out, you see that it flows upwards and as it does, it changes into a pale magenta and then into pure white light. This is the centre which allows us, when we are ready, to be in touch with the spiritual aspect of our being.

Now bring your concentration into the whole of your aura. Feel it vibrating in harmony, being filled with all the clear pure colours of the spectrum. Feel these colours bringing health, vitality and well being into the physical body.

Gently bring your concentration back into your physical body. Be aware of your physical body lying or sitting on the floor. As you become aware of your body, surround it with an orb of beautiful blue light for protection. Gradually, you are going to bring your body back into everyday activity.

Starting with your toes, gently begin to move them. Now gently flex the muscles of your legs, individually and then both together. Slowly start to move your fingers, as if you were playing the piano. Breathing in, bring your arms up over your head, stretching the whole of the body. Exhaling, bring your arms back down to your sides. Repeat this twice more. Gently move your head from side to side. When you are ready open your eyes and feel yourself completely returned to everyday activity. Roll over onto your right-hand side and stand up. Be aware of any differences which have occurred, mentally, physically and spiritually. Take note of these and compare them with your experiences next time you do this relaxation and energising exercise.

CHAKRA MEDITATION

To prepare for this meditation, select a place which is quiet and warm and where you will not be disturbed. Sit either on a chair or on the floor, whichever you find is more comfortable. If you are sitting on a chair, place both feet on the floor with your hands on your knees. This is the pharaoh posture. If you sit on the floor, sit either in the half or full lotus or against a wall with your legs stretched out in front of you and a cushion behind your back. Whichever posture you choose, make sure that the spine is straight and the head, face and neck free from tension.

Gently close your eyes and bring your concentration into the gentle inhalation and exhalation of the breath. As you exhale, breathe out any tension in the physical body. If any part of the body feels uncomfortable change to a more comfortable position. From the breath, move your concentration to the gentle and slow beat of the heart. Now bring that concentration to the spine. Visualise it as a column of light which anchors you to the earth but is also able to lift you up into the spiritual realm. Visualise that column of light as containing seven energy centres, each radiating its own beautiful, ethereal colour. Move down to the base of the spine where you will find the first centre. Standing outside of the base centre, slowly start to walk into it. As you enter, you will see before you the beautiful white bud of a flower. Go up to it and gently touch it. At your touch it starts to open revealing at its centre a red ruby. The rays which emanate from this stone infuse the petals with its colour.

Stepping into this centre of the flower and sitting down by the stone, you are engulfed in this colour. You feel its warmth touching every part of your body. You feel a physical attachment to earth, to its stability and solidarity and you realise that part of you is a physical being. Looking into the centre of the stone you see a narrow shaft of white light reaching upwards. It feels as though it is pulling you to-

140

wards it. Get up and move towards it. On reaching this light you feel it gently lifting you up, lifting you into the second centre.

As you stand in the sacral centre, the beautiful white bud faces you. Gently running your hands over it, you feel its softness. It responds to your touch by opening and revealing at its centre an amber stone. This stone sends out deep pure orange rays which the petals reflect. Stepping into the centre of the flower and sitting down, letting the body be engulfed in this colour, you feel any sadness or depression being lifted from you. You feel as though the whole of your body is being energised and filled with joy and laughter. Looking to the centre of the stone you see the shaft of white light. You arise and walk towards it so that it may lift you up into the third centre.

In the solar plexus centre, stand and look at that white bud. Look at the beauty and perfection of its creation. Touch it with awe and wonder. As it opens, it reveals to you at its centre a yellow topaz. Walk into the flower and sit down by the stone. Immediately you feel a sense of detachment as this colour surrounds you. You feel detached from problems, worries and anxieties. This enables you to see these things more clearly and to put them into perspective. It detaches you from fellow human beings and you realise that each person has to find and follow their own path, whatever that path may bring. With a feeling of gratitude turn towards the shaft of white light, allowing it to lift you gently up into the fourth centre.

As you look at the white bud which is at the heart centre, you suddenly feel great love and respect for it. You express this love through your hands as you touch the outside of its petals. It responds by opening and showing you at its centre a beautiful green emerald which tints its petals with clear green light. As you enter and sit down, you feel your body being cleared of toxins and impurities, and your energies being balanced. You feel your body, mind and spirit being brought into harmony and with this a tremendous feeling of spiritual love surges through you. This love you take with you as you go to the shaft of white light and allow it to lift you up into the fifth or throat centre.

Standing by the white bud, you notice that this centre feels different. You realise that you are on a bridge, the crossing point from the physical into the spiritual realm.

At this point you can turn back if you feel that the time is not right for you to continue. If you feel that it is right, cross this bridge and touch the bud that awaits you with reverence and awe and wait for it to open. As it opens, you find at its centre a dark blue sapphire. The rays reflect on the petals and then lift upwards into the spiritual realm. Entering the flower and sitting at its centre you feel tremendous peace, relaxation and calm. You feel as though you have been lifted out of the earthly environment into a new realm of being. Rest for a while, letting this deep sense of being well up from within you. Feeling the need to move on, once more find the shaft of light and allow it to lift you up into the sixth or brow centre.

Standing at the third-eye centre, gently encase the bud with your hands. Watch it open and reveal to you at its centre a deep violet amethyst. As you walk towards the stone you feel its healing power entering your body, mind and spirit. You feel a sense of dignity with this colour, the dignity that you should have as a human being in all aspects of life. Pondering on this thought you enter the shaft of white light so that it can lift you up into the seventh centre, the crown.

At this centre we find that the flower is already open. Situated at its centre is a many faceted diamond. The rays coming from this stone display all the colours of the spectrum. They dance and play on the petals of the flower making it look multi-coloured. Standing at the centre, look up, and you will see that all of these colours are reflecting upwards and merging into a brilliant white light. Stand and look into this light. Behold the vastness, beauty, love and wonder of the spiritual realm. Stand and reflect on what this means and reveals to you. Stretch out your arms and embrace this light. As you stand with your arms stretched out, into your hands is placed a candle. The flame from this candle sends its light out in all directions. This flame represents all that the spiritual realm reveals to you. Take the flame and encase it safely into your heart, letting it be revealed only to those who are ready to hear. With this precious gift you must now start your journey back into earth consciousness.

Taking a circle of light which encloses a cross of light, you are going back down into the seven centres. Encompass these centres with this circle and cross and watch as the flowers gently close. Starting with the crown centre, encircle the flower with the circle of light which contains the cross of light and watch the flower gently close. Now come down to the brow centre, doing the same, down into the throat centre, the heart centre, the solar plexus centre, the sacral centre and finally the base centre. As you enter this last centre, feel the colour red earthing you and bringing you fully back into earth consciousness. Gently encircle and close this flower. Feeling yourself fully returned, gently open your eyes.

CHANDRA NAMASKARA

SALUTE TO THE MOON

Chandra namaskara, or 'salute to the moon', is the complementary series of movements to surya namaskara (see pp. 31–44). Surya, the sun, represents the male energy, and chandra, the moon, represents the female energy.

Chandra namaskara comprises twenty-four postures which work with the entire physical body. These postures work with every muscle, helping to remove tension, to strengthen and to make supple. In particular, they strengthen and make supple the spine, and tone the spinal nerves.

Originally, these movements were performed at dusk, just as the sun was setting and the moon rising. Whilst practising chandra, one absorbed into one's being the energy which radiated from the moon. The power of this energy depended upon whether the moon was full, waxing or waning, a full moon possessing the most powerful energy. One also thought about the feminine aspect of one's being. Male and female possess both the feminine and masculine energies. If one incarnates into a masculine body, then a female aura surrounds this body. If one has a female body, then a male aura will surround it. Unfortunately, the female energy in a lot of men tends to be suppressed. They are conditioned into thinking that it is not manly to possess sensitivity or to show any kind of emotion. This can create blockages in that person which could manifest as disease.

If one is able to accept these energies and to practise chandra with full knowledge of them, then any blockages which have been created, can be slowly and gently dispersed. This can only happen if a man is prepared to accept the feminine aspect of himself and a woman the masculine aspect. Whilst it is preferable to practise chandra at sunset, for the reasons given above, it is still beneficial when practised at other times during the day.

The movements of chandra namaskara are a little more strenuous then surya, so it is advisable, if you are a beginner, to master the movements of surya before attempting chandra.

Like surya, chandra can be used purely as warming up movements, or, it can be used as a meditation exercise. If it is used as warming up movements, first learn the series of movements and then, when you are familiar with them, add the correct breathing. Used for this purpose, it can be performed as many times as is comfortable, without strain.

When it is used as a meditation exercise, the movements are performed more slowly. Again, it is essential to know the series of movements by heart and not have to keep stopping to look at the book. This is not conducive to a meditative state. For meditation, the awareness is brought firstly into the physical body. One becomes aware of the inhalations and exhalations of the breath. From the breath, move the concentration to the muscles and joints, feeling which ones are being used with each movement. From the muscles and joints one becomes aware of the organs of the body, feeling them being stretched, compressed and toned. From this body awareness, the concentration is centred upon the chakras, which are activated with the postures, and the colours which radiate from these chakras. Visualise these colours flooding into the chakras from the universe, bringing them into harmony and balance. Red, orange and yellow enter the body through the feet. Green enters horizontally into the heart chakra and blue, indigo and violet come in through the top of the head. From the chakras, allow the colour to radiate out into the aura to bring harmony and balance to body, mind and spirit.

To experience the benefits of chandra namaskara on a physical, mental and spiritual level, it must be practised regularly.

1st Position — PRANAMASANA
— Prayer Pose

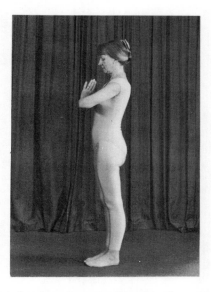

Stand in an upright posture with the feet together and the spine straight. Take the shoulders back and down in order to open the chest. Bring the hands together into the prayer position. Point the thumbs towards the heart chakra to acknowledge the seat of the true self. Relax the whole body, breathing normally. Bring your concentration into the heart centre. Visualise the colour green radiating from this chakra, bringing harmony and balance into the physical body.

2nd Position — HASTA UTTANASANA — Salutation

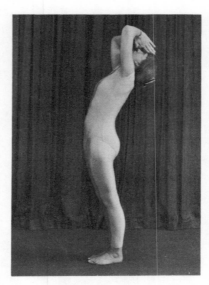

Keeping the hands in the prayer position, inhale and raise the arms over the head until the fingers touch the forehead. At the same time, bend the trunk of the body and the head backwards. Bring your concentration into the throat or vishuddha chakra. Visualise a clear blue radiating out from this chakra bringing peace and relaxation to the physical body.

3rd Position — PADANGUSTHASANA
— Hand-to-foot Posture

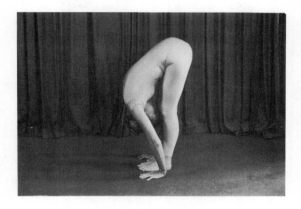

Exhaling, extend the body forward from the hips, making sure that the spine is kept straight. Place the palms of the hands on the floor by the side of the feet with the fingers facing forwards. Keep the knees locked and the hips in line with the ankles. Bring your concentration into the swadhisthana chakra. Visualise a pure orange radiating from this centre bringing energy and joy into every cell of the physical body.

4th Position
— The Lunge

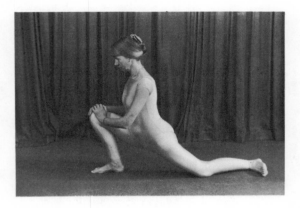

Inhaling, extend the left foot back as far as possible, turning the left foot outwards to make a 90-degree angle with the leg. Place both of the hands on to the right knee. Lift up the trunk of the body and take the shoulders back and down, so that the chest is expanded. Bring your concentration into the ajna chakra and visualise a deep indigo radiating from this centre.

5th Position
— Standing Triangle

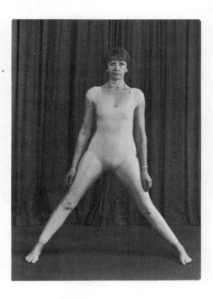

Exhaling, press the hands down onto the right knee and bring the body into standing posture. In this position, the right foot should be facing forwards and the left foot should be turned outwards, forming a right angle with the right foot. Turn the body and the right foot to the left to form the standing triangle. Make sure that the feet are parallel, with the toes in line with each other. The spine should be straight and the shoulders taken back and down. Bring your concentration into the heart centre. Let the green from this chakra radiate out into the aura, bringing harmony and balance into the body.

6th Position — ASHWA SANCHALANASANA — Equestrian Posture

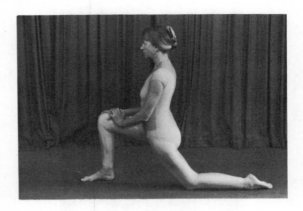

Inhaling, turn both of the feet and the body to the right. Bend both knees so that the left knee rests on the floor and the right knee forms a right angle with the right leg. Make sure that the right knee is vertically in line with the ankle. Rest the hands on the right knee. Bring your concentration into the ajna chakra. Visualise a deep indigo flooding this centre and then radiating out into the aura.

7th Position
— Half Moon Posture

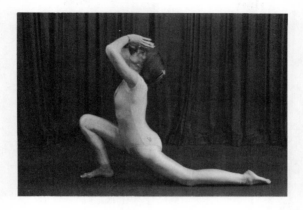

Exhale, and on the next inhalation, bring the hands into the prayer position. Raise the arms and hands over the head until the fingers touch the forehead. At the same time, bend the trunk of the body and the head back. Bring your concentration into the vishuddha or throat chakra. Visualise a clear blue flooding and radiating out from this centre, giving a feeling of peace and tranquillity.

8th Position — ADHO MUKHA SVANASANA — Dog Posture

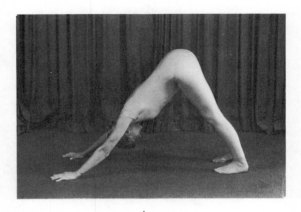

Exhaling, and keeping the hands in the prayer position, move the head and trunk forward and down, until it rests on the right knee. Then take the hands down and place them on either side of the right foot. Straighten the left leg and take the right leg back to join it. Keeping both feet on the floor and the arms and spine straight, press down with the hands in order to bring the head as near to the floor as possible. Concentrate on the swadisthana chakra and visualise a pure orange radiating out from this centre bringing joy and energy into the whole of the physical body.

9th Position
— Raised Cobra

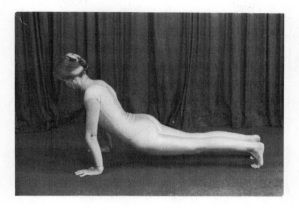

On the next inhalation, keeping the arms straight, gently lower the body until the legs are parallel with the floor. Press the abdomen towards the floor in order to lift up the head and trunk into the raised cobra position. Make sure that the shoulders are back and down, to encourage the opening of the chest and to ensure that the neck is free from tension. The completed posture is supported entirely by the hands and toes. Bring your awareness into the manipura or solar plexus chakra. Allow the yellow to radiate out from this centre, bringing detachment from any problems or worries that may be present.

10th Position — ADHO MUKHA SVANASANA — Dog Posture

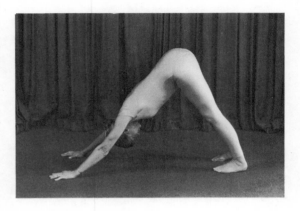

Exhaling, press down with the hands and raise the buttocks in order to come back into the dog posture. Keep the feet on the floor and the legs and the spine straight. Continue to press down with the hands to allow the head to come as near as possible to the floor. Again bring your concentration into the swadisthana chakra. Feel the energy and joy that this orange colour gives.

11th Position
— The Lunge

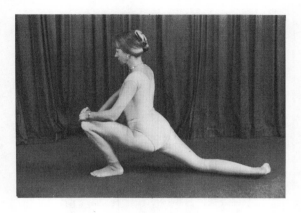

Inhaling, bring the left foot forward and place it between the hands. Bend both of the knees, so that the right knee rests on the floor, with the right foot turned outwards to make a 90-degree angle with the right leg. The left knee is in a vertical line with the left ankle. Lift up the spine and raise the hands on to the left knee. Extend the left knee slightly forwards. The shoulders are taken back and down in order to open out the chest. Bring your awareness into the ajna chakra and the indigo which radiates from it.

12th Position
— Standing Triangle

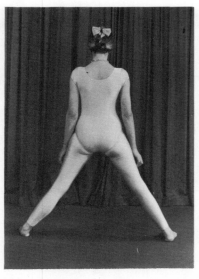

Exhaling, press down on the left knee and bring the body into the standing posture. In this position, the left foot should be facing forwards and the right foot turned outwards to form a right angle with the left foot. Now turn the body and the left foot to the right to form the standing triangle. Make sure that the feet are parallel, with the toes in line with each other. The spine should be straight and the shoulders taken back in order to open the chest. Bring your concentration into the heart chakra and the green which radiates from it. Allow this colour to bring the negative and positive energies of the body into balance.

13th Position — ASHWA SANCHALANASANA
— Equestrian Posture

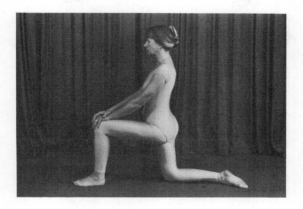

Inhaling, turn both of the feet and the body to the left. Bend both of the knees, resting the right knee and the top of the right foot on the floor, and forming a right angle with the left knee. Make sure that the left knee is vertically in line with the ankle. Rest the hands on the left knee. Bring your concentration back to the ajna chakra and the deep indigo which radiates from it.

14th Position
— Half Moon Posture

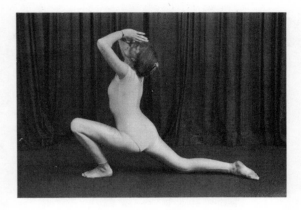

Exhale, and bring the hands into the prayer position. Inhaling, raise the arms and hands over the head until the fingers touch the forehead. At the same time, bend the trunk of the body and the head back. Bring the concentration back to the vishuddhi or throat chakra and the clear blue colour which radiates from it.

15th Position — ADHO MUKHA SVANASANA — Dog Posture

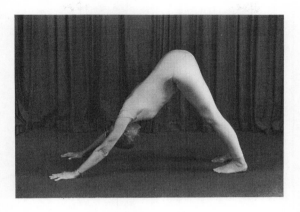

Exhaling, and keeping the hands in the prayer position, move the head and trunk forward and down until it rests on the left knee. Then take the hands down and place them on either side of the left foot, with the fingers pointing forwards. Straighten the right leg and take the left leg back to join it. Keep both of the feet flat on the floor and the arms and spine straight. Press down with the hands and raise the buttocks into the air, allowing the head to come as near to the floor as possible. Bring your awareness into the swadisthana chakra and the pure orange colour which radiates from it.

16th Position
— Raised Cobra

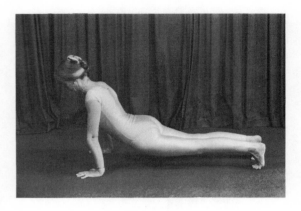

On the next inhalation, keeping the arms straight, gently lower the body until the legs are parallel with the floor. Press the abdomen towards the floor in order to lift up the head and trunk into the raised cobra position. Make sure that the shoulders are back and down, to open the chest and to release the neck. Bring your awareness into the manipura chakra and the pure yellow colour which radiates from it.

17th Position — ADHO MUKHA SVANASANA — Dog Posture

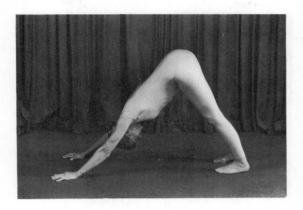

Exhaling, press down with the hands and raise the buttocks in order to come back into the dog posture. Remember to keep the feet on the floor and the legs and spine straight. Continue to press down with the hands to allow the head to come as near to the floor as is possible. Bring your concentration back into the swadisthana chakra. Feel this colour and the energy and joy that it gives.

18th Position — SHASHANKASANA
— The Pose of the Moon

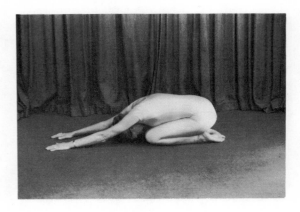

Inhaling, bend both of the knees down to the floor. Place the toes flat and sit back on the heels. Exhaling, bend the body forward to rest on the thighs, bringing the forehead on to the floor. Make sure that the buttocks remain in contact with the heels. Stretch the arms out in front of the body with the palms of the hands on the floor. Bring your concentration into the base or muladhara chakra. Visualise the colour red radiating out from this centre. Feel it bringing vitality to the body and earthing you to this planet.

19th Position
— New Moon Posture

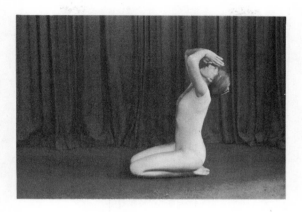

Still sitting on the heels, inhale and raise the body to the vertical position. At the same time, bring the hands into the prayer position. Gently bend the body back and raise the arms and hands over the head until the fingers come into contact with the forehead. Bring the concentration into the vishuddha chakra and feel what effect the colour blue has on you as it radiates from this centre out into the aura.

20th Position
— Raised Cobra

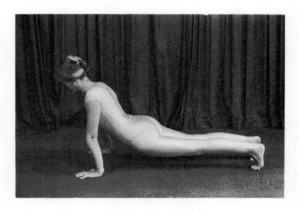

Exhaling, bring the trunk of the body forward and raise the buttocks from the heels. Place the hands, fingers facing forwards, onto the floor, so that they are in line with the knees and form a straight line with the shoulders.

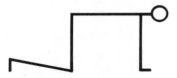

Inhaling, making sure that the arms are kept straight, tuck the toes of both feet under and straighten the legs until they are parallel with the floor. Gently lower the abdomen towards the floor in order to lift up the head and trunk into the raised cobra. Make sure that the shoulders are taken down and back in order to open the chest and release the neck. Bring your concentration into the manipura chakra. Feel the colour yellow as it radiates out from this centre and try to be aware of its effect on the physical, mental and spiritual bodies.

21st Position — ADHO MUKHA SVANASANA — Dog Posture

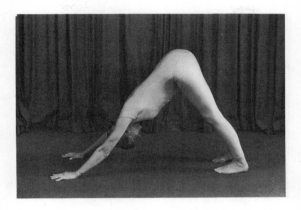

Exhaling, press down with the hands and raise the buttocks up. Keep pressing down with the hands in order to bring the head as near to the floor as possible. Bring the concentration into the swadisthana chakra. Feel the orange colour as it radiates out from this centre and feel what effect it has upon your whole being.

22nd Position
— Squat Posture

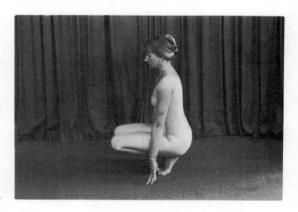

Inhaling, raise the head and jump both feet forward to land between and level with both hands. Raise the hands onto the fingertips. Bring your awareness into the ajna chakra. Feel the indigo colour which radiates from this centre and the effect which it has on the whole being.

23rd Position — PADANGUSTHASANA
— Hand-to-foot Posture

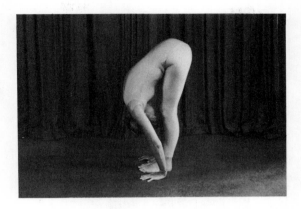

Exhaling, lower the hands onto the floor by the side of the feet. Press down with the hands and straighten the legs, keeping the trunk of the body and the head as close to the legs as possible. In this position, make sure that the knees are kept locked, that the hips are in line with the ankles and the spine is straight. Bring your concentration into the swadisthana chakra. Feel the colour of orange which radiates from it and the joy and energy which it gives.

24th Position — PRANAMASANA
— Prayer Posture

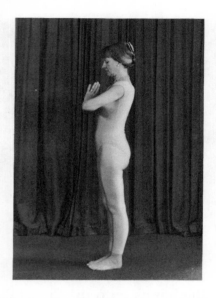

Inhaling, unfold the body back to the standing posture. Bring the hands together into the prayer position, with the thumbs pointing towards the heart centre. Check that the feet are together, the spine straight and the chest opened. Bring your awareness into the heart centre and feel the spiritual love which radiates from this centre, radiating out to all living things upon this planet earth.

THE THREE HIGHER CHAKRAS

We have, through many deep discussions, accompanied by loving questioning, found that there are at least three higher chakras above the crown chakra. The pages that follow, describe what we have discovered in the magenta, the white, and the ultimate chakra. Because these chakras are in the early stages of recognition, we cannot, as yet, give complete visualisations for them. You may, however, like to meditate on what we have been able to realise, and each person may individually discover more of their individual meaning.

MAGENTA, The Chakra of the Higher Self

When the higher self enters into being and completely illuminates every cell with almost white light, the colour which appears is red turned into magenta. The red, which no longer wants to be the power, becomes the complete service of love.

Magenta, or peach blossom, is the colour of the completed higher self. It shines into the physical being but is not of the physical. Such a being has balanced out all its forces and thereby can state, 'Not of me but through me shines the unlimited love. This has not been demanded of me, but I am offering it through me because it is the ultimate freedom of free will.'

This will has no other direction except to love. Mankind was chosen to do this for the whole of the angelic hierarchies so that they in turn can achieve it.

We can also say that this is a chakra completely outside the body, but attainable and potentially available to all human beings.

The Meaning of the Colour Magenta

Both priest and priestess have accepted the dignified divinity and have risen above the state of only service. They now enter the state of the creator. It is at this stage that the red of love completely envelops the clear and beautiful violet and creates this colour of magenta, the colour of spirit and of utmost purity.

All intentions to act out of my own limitations have left and I now act out of unlimited and undemanded love. We have learned that no other power will serve. The state of freedom has come. We have decided not to decide but to let the original creational force work through us. We still have a free will which can oppose this force. But we realise that to oppose it causes negativity. The challenger, who ultimately led us to this point, has also fulfilled its own purpose by giving us the choice to be free or enslaved. At the time of the creation (which is at any moment, and out of time and space), there stands the reality of life and the truth of knowledge. This knowledge enables us to understand life. The two principles must cooperate with each other. Having experienced the energies of all the colours, we have lost sight of the oneness out of which they originated. This source was the principle of life. Knowledge can no longer stand on its own, it must now support life. When it does this, it is the colour of magenta which builds the arch between knowledge and life. In the magenta, the human being is seen to use this bridge, which is built of pure love alone. This knowledge and life create a new trinity: Love — Truth — Life.

Meditation with the Colour Magenta

The previous colour, violet, has already guided me into a spiritual concept of myself. Magenta in its luminous almost white form, is the ultimate colour to let go of all that relates to little me, the little me which wants, needs, has to have, craves for and wants to impress.

Magenta, the inner colour of the ultimate illumination beyond which we cannot comprehend anything except complete, absolute, unlimited, undemanding awareness of all thoughts, feelings and life essences. The purest invisible energy. The most perfect love which has no other purpose than to let all be in its most beautiful perfection. The power of love which does not use its power, but thereby remains the source of eternal life.

Let go. Just be. Let time and space dissolve. I am aware that this absolute void becomes the point where a new me can be found. I let all thoughts slip away. They become a part of a firm foundation upon which I can now stand safely. I make this my stepping stone. There is now a moment of no thing. Out of this comes a most exquisite fine and pure shining magenta. It is like silver shining out of space. It comes towards me, and yet I am in it. My inner gaze is guided to see a perfect human being and as the image becomes clearer, I recognise myself, not as I am now, but as I shall be when I have attained that complete status of my higher self. Why do I see this image now? I seem to open my lips and say, 'I am a part of the plan which always was, is now and will be.'

I do not have to ask what part I have to be. I am aware that I am where I need to be now. I always was there, but faced with a multitude of things around me, I eventually could not see that place and put many unnecessary obstacles in the way. Now these are no longer obstacles but stepping stones. I go from one to the next, and realise that I am who I am and bring the message I always intended to bring. I now know the infinite knowledge and know that I do not need to use this. I am used because the universe knows that I know, and in this selfless state I am now pure energy. I am where I am the perfect part of the whole. Perfect peace. Love without self.

Retaining this knowledge and experience, slowly start to return to everyday consciousness.

Visualisation on the Colour Magenta

Calmly and peacefully relax. Search in your mind to find that magenta colour which connects itself to your thoughts, feelings and images.

When you read the section on the meaning of the colour magenta, ask yourself which part made the strongest impression. Now try and make a strong but steady image by looking into the magenta colour. Strengthen it, focus into this colour and collect and feel its energy.

Change is one of its energies, but also to become objective about your own self is another. Let go of all that has been holding you back. Magenta is also the colour which points into the future.

WHITE, The Higher Chakra of Consciousness

At the point where all colour has dissolved into the pure white spirit, we receive a light which appears without colour. The white contains all and at the same time contains nothing because it has never absorbed any density or weight. It is the result of all things which have been overcome by us. It has carried us through the darkness, the darkness which has never denied or destroyed it. The darkness has protected the white light to the point where it took its dark mantle so that those who cannot as yet see it, would not have to endure suffering.

The darkness loves the white light so much that it gave it all the experiences which it needed to absorb. Now it rises out of this long vast energy of loving teaching, loving

174

protection, loving embrace of experience with greater purity, greater consciousness and with greater protection because of the knowledge that it is now the only force of the spirit which can never be destroyed. Because it knows this and also knows the last secret, when the time is right, this knowledge will be bestowed upon all beings. It once made itself vulnerable, so as to partake in all events which contained all possible possibilities. Now it has risen into the purest of all pure existence on the spiral of colour and music, on the evolutionary chain of all events. White, the everlasting innocence, which can never fall because it has risen out of experience to its higher origin. It did not know at the journey's outset that there was a purer innocence. Now it is white.

Meditation on White

I am standing on the edge of the purest new fallen snow. The morning mist has not yet dispersed and the sun, just risen, glows through the pure white atmosphere in which I am standing. I have gathered all my own being to the point where I am sure of my place, my time and my task. Without these three affirmations, I could not now stand at this last challenge. I am here to find myself, to find that which I am meant to be, so that I can be a tool for God. I allow to sink down into the world out of which I have just stepped, all strange, unnecessary and even plaguing thoughts. Let go; these are no longer important. Let go. I can be free at this time and let timelessness take over. To be in white is now all I need, all I want, all I wish to experience.

The snow is still new. The mist gradually disperses and drifts to a lower place where it joins lovingly with the river of life. I now stand facing the one way. I am given my direction, knowing that I can say thank you for this guidance which will place me where I can be the best servant in the plan of life.

I turn with this thought, back to the planet and remember my task, to be the tool of God. I remember this when I return back into all the colours of the world. The world in which I have chosen to be.

White, I will take you into this world of colour where I want to make all colours fill with your power. I can find my way back to this beautiful place when I need to be replenished with your life force.

Return back to the place where you are meditating, and to your daily work, but remember, that this source of life is always at your disposal.

Visualisation and Awareness on White

No colour is all colours, so luminous that the human perception can only recognise this as white.

In a white environment we can stay only for a comparatively short time, otherwise we become so detached that we might become insecure.

Place yourself into the three dimensional space of the room in which you are sitting. Feel the space. Become fully aware of the length of the room, the width and the height. Now look on a pure white surface, such as a white curtain or a white rose, and then close your eyes. White represents purity, innocence, newness. Since all of these are remote from the modern person, you need to let all past events and experiences sink gently below you into the foundation, represented by the floor on which you now sit. Look at all things which have involved you, as if these have happened to some good friend of yours. Look at them with detachment, without any emotional ties. All is now slipping into the foundation which is like solid but absorbent clay.

Start first with present happenings. Maybe today or yesterday. Then go back a few days, then back to last week, last month, last year. Go back as far as your memory will let you. Gradually all the events have been allowed to go away, and you can say thank you for this. All the colours which were present in those events are also gone. Only the white remains.

In this pure and beautiful white, a silver figure appears before your inner eyes. Ask this being to help you to reach into this realm where there is no judgement, no blame nor any shame. All that I am today is due to these past experiences which I have had to go through in order to arrive here in this white state of purity. Anything that I wish to undertake out of this pure new state is pure and new, only supported by the wisdom which I have gathered so far on my path through life.

THE ULTIMATE CHAKRA

From out of the sacred darkness,
came light.
The union of light and darkness,
brought forth colour.
From colour came sound.
From sound form.
But all contain and come from
this original sacred darkness.

In the state of pure, absolute existence, where all forces of life, love and light take their origin, there was no origin. There never was a beginning because on the eternal spiral there can never be an ending. This force of love which has no demands, which has no limits, just is. It did not know a name by which to call itself. It had no place to place itself and did not know its own face. The holy or the whole darkness which stands at the ultimate point, is the cradle out of which all is born, the womb of eternal creation wherein is contained all that was, is and ever will be. It is the deepest of all colours because it has overcome all needs to be itself; thereby it is all and at the same time the ultimate archetypal mother. Experience of all and innocence of nothing. Sacred colourless black which is neither negative nor positive but which is because it is.

PRACTICE SESSION FOR A BEGINNER

Read the instructions for all the postures which have been given in this example lesson before you start to practise them. Perform each posture twice. When you perform the posture the first time, your concentration should be on the physical body. This enables you to check that each part of your body is correctly placed and to discover which joints and muscles are being used, and which organs are being activated. This will help you to get to know and understand how your body functions. When you repeat the posture, your concentration should be centred on the relevant chakra and the colour which radiates from it. If you are uncertain as to where the chakras are located, look at the diagrams on pages 18 and 20.

1 Start your session with a short relaxation as given for the advanced student. See page 181.

2 *Prasarita Padottasana*. Pages 126–7.
   Whilst holding this posture, bring your concentration into the crown chakra. Visualise a ray of bright violet light coming from the universe into this centre. If your concentration starts to wander, gently bring it back. Now see if you can make this colour extend out from the chakra into your aura.

3 *Ardha Matsyendrasana* (Half abdominal twist). Pages 118–19.
   Whilst holding this posture, bring your concentration into the ajna or brow chakra. Visualise a ray of indigo

light coming through the top of your head and flooding this centre. Before extending this colour into your aura, try to feel what effect it has upon this chakra.

4 *Ardha Chandrasana* (The crescent moon pose). Pages 109–10.
When holding this posture, bring your concentration into the throat or vishuddha chakra. Visualise a ray of clear blue light coming through the top of your head and into this centre. Try to be aware of the peace, tranquillity and relaxation that this colour gives you. Gently start to visualise the colour expanding out into your aura.

5 *Matsyasana* (Fish pose). — Variation 1. Pages 88–9.
Whilst holding this posture, bring a ray of bright green light horizontally into the heart or anahata chakra. If any part of your being feels out of balance, feel this colour restoring it to harmony. Now expand this colour from the chakra out into the aura.

6 *Bhujangasana* (The cobra). Page 39.
When you have checked that each part of your body is positioned correctly, bring a shaft of yellow light through the soles of your feet, into the solar plexus or manipura chakra. Try to allow this colour to detach your thoughts from any slight discomfort which you may be experiencing. Gradually start to radiate this colour out into your aura.

7 *Padangusthasana* (Hand-to-foot pose). Page 35.
Allow your body to relax slowly into this posture. When in the posture, bring your awareness into the sacral or swadisthana chakra. Visualise a shaft of orange light coming through the soles of your feet into this centre. Let this colour fill you with joy and happiness, removing any depression or sadness which you may have. Now visualise this colour radiating out into your aura.

8 *The arm-leg-link*. Page 53.
When you have mastered your balance in this posture, bring your concentration into the base or muladhara chakra. Visualise a bright clear red coming through the earth and into this centre. Feel this colour grounding you to the earth and providing your body with the correct amount of warmth for its needs. Gradually extend this colour out into your aura. As you sit in this posture, see yourself clothed in a coat of bright, shimmering, dancing colours. Each one is in harmony with the others.

9 Select one of the colours which you have been working with and practise the awareness exercise given for this colour.

10 Read about the meaning of the colour which you have selected.

11 To finish, either practise the meditation for your chosen colour or end with a relaxation which you will find on page 24.

PRACTICE SESSION FOR AN ADVANCED STUDENT

Start your session by lying on the floor for five minutes in savāsana, (the corpse posture). During this time, try to detach your mind from any thoughts. Visualise these thoughts as beautiful bubbles which float up into the atmosphere and then gently disperse. When your mind has become calm and peaceful, bring your concentration into your physical body. Feel each part of your body for any tension. Start with your head and work down your body to your feet. Gently let go of any tension and feel yourself starting to relax. It is much easier to go into a posture with relaxed muscles than with ones which are in tension. When you have released as much tension from your body as you can, spend a few moments in this relaxed state. On the next inhalation, bring your arms up over your head and stretch your whole body. Exhaling, bring your arms back down to your side. Repeat this twice more, then gently roll over onto your side and sit up.

1 Perform three rounds of surya or chandra namaskara as a warming up exercise. At the end of these rounds, go into the pose of a child and relax. During this short relaxation feel what effect this has had on you.

2 *Sirasana* (Head balance). Pages 129–31.
Whilst holding this posture, bring your concentration into the crown chakra. Visualise a shaft of pure violet light coming from the universe, through the top of your

head and into this centre. Visualise any blockages being released before you allow this colour to radiate out into your aura. As it radiates out, watch as it rises above your head and changes into a pale magenta, the colour of the higher self. When you come down from this posture, relax for a few minutes.

3 *Gomukhasana* (The cowhead posture). Pages 115–16.
When you are in this posture, bring a shaft of indigo light through the top of your head into the ajna chakra. Allow this light to bring this centre into harmony and balance before radiating out into the aura. Work with this posture on both sides of the body and then relax for a few minutes.

4 *Sarvangasana* (The shoulder balance). Pages 107–8.
When holding this posture, bring your concentration into the throat centre. Visualise a shaft of pure blue light coming through the top of your head into this chakra, bringing it into harmony and balance. Feel the sense of peace and tranquillity that this colour gives you when it radiates out into your aura. As soon as you start to feel tired, bring your legs down into halasana (the plough, pp. 105–6). Continue to concentrate on the throat centre. Finally come into savāsana (corpse posture) and relax.

5 *Matsyasana* (The fish posture). Pages 88–9.
In this posture, visualise a shaft of pure green entering horizontally the anahata or heart chakra. Feel this colour not only bringing this centre into balance, but also balancing the positive and negative energies in your body. As it radiates out into your aura it brings your body, mind and spirit into harmony to make you a whole being. This centre is the centre of spiritual love. If for any reason you are suffering from a 'broken heart', you can bring a shaft of amethyst light into this chakra. This colour has tremendous healing power. This should be

followed with rose pink, the colour of spiritual love. Once this chakra has been healed with amethyst, it should be filled with the rose pink of spiritual love.

6 *Uttana Mayurasana* (The bridge). Pages 80–1.
Whilst holding this posture, visualise a shaft of pure yellow light coming through the soles of your feet, into the manipura or solar plexus chakra. With the stress and strain of modern living, this chakra is frequently out of balance. As the yellow enters this centre, feel it detaching you from any problems or worries which you may have. If we allow ourselves to become detached, frequently we can look at our problems in a new light and see more clearly the solutions to them. When this colour has flooded the solar plexus chakra, visualise it flowing out into your aura.

7 *Paschimottanasana* (The back-stretching pose). Page 63.
When going into this posture, take it slowly in order to give your body time to relax into it. Whilst holding the posture, bring a shaft of pure orange light through the soles of your feet into the swadisthana chakra. Experience the joy and vitality of this colour. Let this vitality permeate every cell of your being and let the joy dissolve any depression or negative feelings that you have.

8 *Padmasana* (Full lotus posture). Page 54.
Sitting quietly in this posture, bring your concentration into the base chakra. Visualise a shaft of clear red light coming through the earth into this centre. Feel the warmth and the energy of creation that this colour has. Watching, as it radiates out into your aura, feel it grounding you firmly to the earth. Still sitting in this posture, be aware of the whole of your being. Try to be aware of any changes which have taken place through practising these postures. Feel your aura pulsating with the colours of the spectrum, each one in perfect harmony and balance.

9 Select a colour that you feel drawn to. Practise the awareness exercise given for this colour.

10 Read the meaning of the colour which you have chosen.

11 Now practise the meditation given for this colour.

12 You can either end this session with the meditation or follow this with a relaxation which you will find on page 24.

Whilst holding the postures, the visualisation of colour can be changed to visualisation of the yantras.

FURTHER READING

Chocron, Daya Sarai, *Healing With Crystals and Gemstones*, Samuel Weiser Inc., 1986.

Gimbel, Theo., *Healing Through Colour*, C.W. Daniel Co., 1980.

Gimbel, Theo., *Key, Lock and Door: Healing and Meditation*, Hygeia Publications, 1976.

Gimbel, Theo., *Form, Sound, Colour and Healing*, C.W. Daniel Co., 1987.

Iyengar, B.K.S., *Light On Yoga*, Mandala Books, George Allen & Unwin Ltd., 1971.

Murti, Krishna, *Meditations*, Victor Gollancz Ltd., 1980.

Saraswati, Swami Satyananda, *Asana, Pranayama Mudra, Bandha*, Bihar School of Yoga, India, 1969.

Saraswati, Swami Satyananda, *Yoga Nidra*, Bihar School of Yoga, India, 1976.

How To Know God — The Yoga Aphorisms of Patanjali, trs. by Swami Prabhavananda and Christopher Isherwood, A Mentor Book, New English Library.

The Bhagavad Gita, Penguin Classic, 1962.

The Dhammapada, Penguin Classic, 1963.

INDEX

If you have enjoyed reading this book, other titles in the Llewellyn/Quantum list will be of interest. These include:

Psychic Sense: Training and Developing Psychic Sensitivity
by Mary Swainson & Louisa Bennett

Seeds of Magick: An Expose' of Modern Occult Practices
by Catherine Summers & Julian Vayne

The Survival Papers: Applied Jungian Psychology
by Daryl Sharp

Exploring the Fourth Dimension: Secrets of the Paranormal
by John Ralphs

The Dream Lover: Transforming Relationships Through Dreams
by Les Peto

In Defense of Astrology: Astrology's Answers to Its Critics
by Robert Parry

Love Spells: Creative Techniques for Magical Relationships
by James Lynn Page

Applied Visualization: A Mind-Body Program
by James Lynn Page

Earth Memory: Sacred Sites—Doorways into Earth's Mysteries
by Paul Devereux

Dowsing for Health: The Applications & Methods for Holistic Healing
by Arthur Bailey

Life Cycles: The Astrology of Inner Space & Its Application to the Rhythms of Life
by Bill Anderton

Ask your bookseller for full details on the complete range of Llewellyn/Quantum titles, or write to the publisher, Llewellyn Publications, P.O. Box 64383, St. Paul, MN 55164-0383.

THE WORKSHEETS

Refer to page 15 for 'Working With The Worksheets'.

An appropriate colour illustration, associated with each programme of exercises, will be found on the *reverse* of each worksheet. These images can be used in meditation.

WORKSHEET NO. 1

Working with red. You will need for this session a red flower in a vase of water.

Refer to page 15 for 'Working With The Worksheets'.

1 Read the meaning of the colour red. Page 46

2 Start with a simple relaxation. Page 24

3 Acquaint yourself with the positions of the chakras. Page 18

4 Perform two rounds of Surya Namaskara (use as an awareness and warming up exercise). Page 31

5 *ASANAS* Whilst holding these postures, bring your awareness into the relevant chakra and try to visualise the colour which radiates from it.

a) Prasarita Paddottanasana (Crown centre) Page 126
b) Nataraja Asana (Brow centre) Page 116
c) Supta Virasana (Throat centre) Page 68
d) Virabhadrasana 1 (Heart centre) Page 91
e) Purvottanasana (Solar plexus centre) Page 77
f) Padangusthasana (Sacral centre) Page 66
g) The Knee Lock (Base centre) Page 50

6 Repeat the Knee Lock. Again visualise the colour red radiating from the base chakra.

7 Visualisation and awareness exercise on the colour red. Page 48

8 Meditation with the colour red. Page 57

9 General Relaxation No. 1. During this relaxation, be aware of any changes or experiences that may have taken place. Page 24

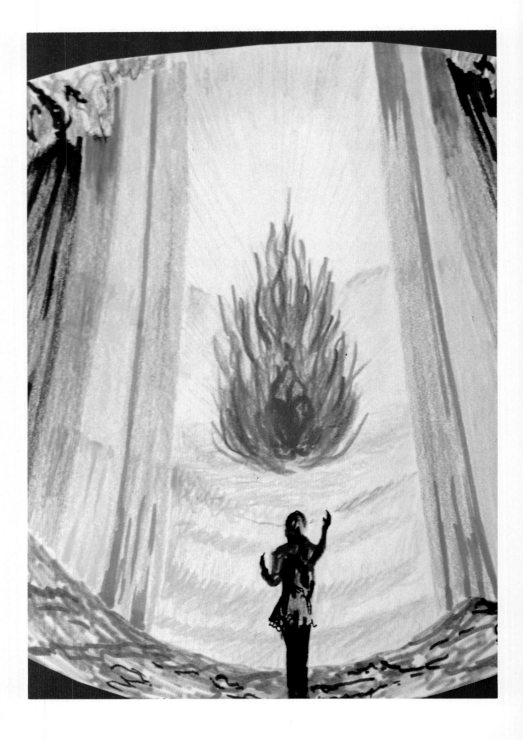

WORKSHEET NO. 2

Working with orange. You will need for this session a piece of carnelian.

1 Read the meaning of the colour orange. Page 60

2 Start with a simple relaxation. Page 24

3 Acquaint yourself with the positions of the chakras. Page 18

4 Perform two rounds of Surya Namaskara. (use as an awareness and warming up exercise). Page 31

5 *ASANAS* Whilst holding these postures, bring your awareness into the relevant chakra and try to visualise the colour which radiates from it.

a) Prasarita Padottanasana (Crown centre)   Page 126
b) Ardha Matsyendrasana (Brow centre)   Page 118
c) Supta Virasana (Throat centre)   Page 68
d) Virabhadrasana 1 (Heart centre)   Page 91
e) Purvottanasana (Solar plexus centre)   Page 77
f) Padangusthasana (Sacral centre)   Page 66
g) The Knee Lock (Base centre)   Page 50

6 Repeat Padangusthasana. Again visualise the colour orange radiating from the sacral centre.

7 Visualisation and awareness exercise on the colour orange. Page 61

8 Meditation with the colour orange. Page 71

9 General Relaxation No. 1. During this relaxation, be aware of any changes or experiences that may have taken place. Page 24

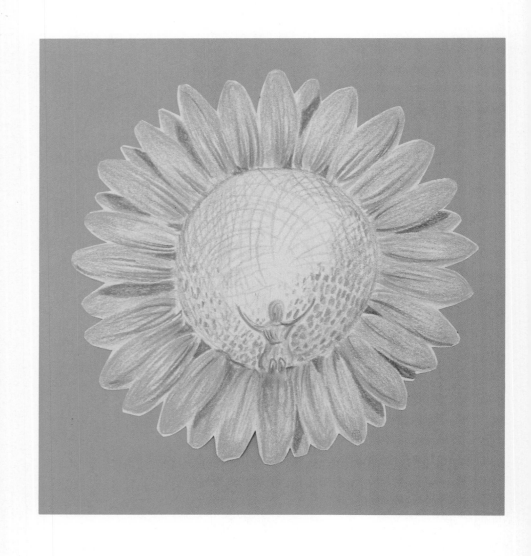

WORKSHEET NO. 3

Working with yellow. You will need for this session a piece of yellow material, either silk or cotton, which is 2 metres long and 1 metre wide.

1 Read the meaning of the colour yellow.   Page 74

2 Start with a simple relaxation.   Page 24

3 Acquaint yourself with the positions of the
  chakras.   Page 18

4 Perform two rounds of Surya Namaskara.
  With each position, visualise the relevant
  chakra.   Page 31

5 *ASANAS* Whilst holding these postures,
          bring your awareness into the relevant
          chakra, visualising the colour which
          radiates from it.

  a) Prasarita Padottanasana (Crown centre)   Page 126
  b) Nataraja Asana (Brow centre)   Page 116
  c) Supta Virasana (Throat centre)   Page 68
  d) Virabhadrasana 2 (Heart centre)   Page 92
  e) Ustrasana (Solar plexus centre)   Page 77
  f) Janu Sirasana (Sacral centre)   Page 64
  g) The Arm Leg Link (Base centre)   Page 53

6 Repeat Ustrasana, visualising yellow flowing
  from the solar plexus chakra.

7 Visualisation and awareness exercise on the
  colour yellow.   Page 75

8 Meditation with the colour yellow.   Page 82

9 General Relaxation No. 1. During this relaxation
  be aware of any changes or experiences that
  you may have had.   Page 24

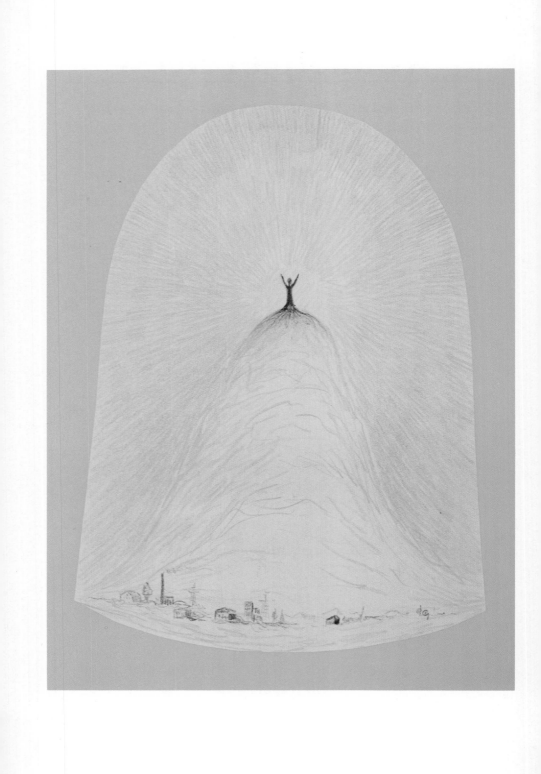

WORKSHEET NO. 4

Working with green. You will need for this session a piece of malachite.

1 Read the meaning of the colour green. Page 85

2 Start with a simple relaxation. Page 24

3 Acquaint yourself with the positions of the chakras. Page 18

4 Perform two rounds of Surya Namaskara. With each position, visualise the relevant chakra. Page 31

5 *ASANAS* Whilst holding these postures, bring your awareness into the relevant chakra and try to visualise the colour which radiates from it.

   a) Bhumi Pada Mastakasana (Crown centre) Page 127
   b) Supta Vajrasana (Throat centre) Page 67
   c) Ardha Matsyendrasana (Brow centre) Page 118
   d) Virabhadrasana 2 (Heart centre) Page 92
   e) Ustrasana (Solar plexus centre) Page 77
   f) Janu Sirasana and Upavistha Konasana (Sacral centre) Pages 64, 65
   g) The Arm Leg Link (Base centre) Page 53

6 Repeat Virabhadrasana 2, visualising green from the heart chakra.

7 Visualisation and awareness exercise on the colour green. Page 86

8 Meditation with the colour green. Page 96

9 General Relaxation No. 1. During this relaxation be aware of any changes or experiences that you may have had. Page 24

199

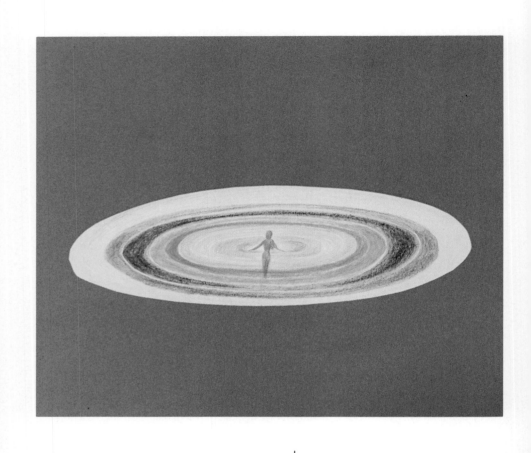

WORKSHEET NO. 5

Working with blue. You will need for this session a blue flower in a vase of water.

1 Read the meaning of the colour blue.   Page 102

2 Start with a simple relaxation.   Page 24

3 Perform three rounds of Surya Namaskara.
   With each position, visualise the relevant
   chakra.   Page 31

4 *ASANAS* Whilst holding these postures,
                bring your awareness into the relevant
                chakra and try to visualise the colour which
                radiates from it.

   a) Bhumi Pada Mastakasana (Crown centre)   Page 127
   b) Gomukhasana (Brow centre)   Page 115
   c) Supta Vajrasana (Throat centre)   Page 67
   d) Matsyasana (Variation 1 or 2) (Heart centre) Page 88
   e) Uttana Mayurasana (Solar plexus centre)   Page 80
   f) Janu Sirasana and Paschimottanasana
       (Sacral centre)   Pages 64, 63
   g) Ardha Navasana 1 (Base centre)   Page 51

5 Repeat Supta Vajrasana, visualising the
   colour blue radiating from the throat centre.

6 Visualisation and awareness exercise on the
   colour blue.   Page 103

7 Meditation with the colour blue.   Page 110

8 General Relaxation No. 2. During this
   relaxation, be aware of any changes or experiences
   you may have had.   Page 27

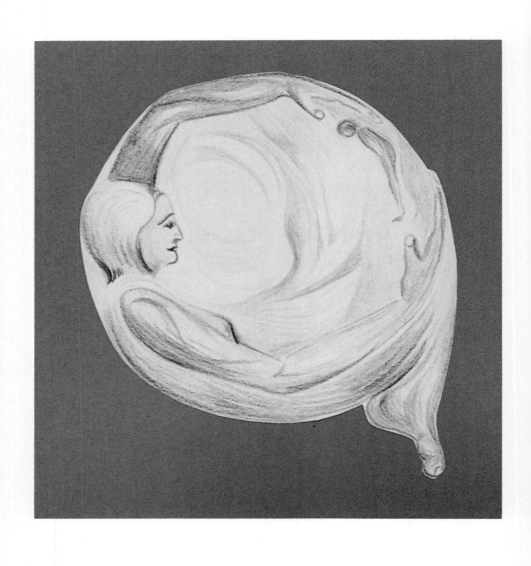

WORKSHEET NO. 6

Working with indigo. You will need a sheet of plain paper, a paintbrush, some indigo and white paint, and the picture of the ajna yantra on the back of this worksheet.

1 Read the meaning of the colour indigo.   Page 112

2 Start with a simple relaxation.   Page 24

3 Perform three rounds of Surya Namaskara.
  With each position, visualise the relevant chakra
  and the colour which radiates from it.   Page 31

4 *ASANAS* Whilst holding these postures,
          bring your awareness into the relevant
          chakra and try to visualise the colour
          which radiates from it.

   a) Bhumi Pada Mastakasana (Crown centre)   Page 127
   b) Nataraja Asana (Brow centre)   Page 116
   c) Ardha Chandrasana (Throat centre)   Page 109
   d) Matsyasana (Variation 1 or 2) (Heart centre) Page 88
   e) Uttana Mayurasana (Solar plexus centre)   Page 80
   f) Janu Sirasana and Paschimottanasana
      (Sacral centre)   Pages 64, 63
   g) Ardha Navasana 2 (Base centre)   Page 51

5 Repeat Nataraja asana, visualising the colour
  indigo radiating from the brow centre.

6 Visualisation and awareness exercise on the
  colour indigo.   Page 113

7 Meditation with the colour indigo.   Page 119

8 General Relaxation No. 2. During this relaxation
  be aware of any changes or experiences you
  may have had.   Page 27

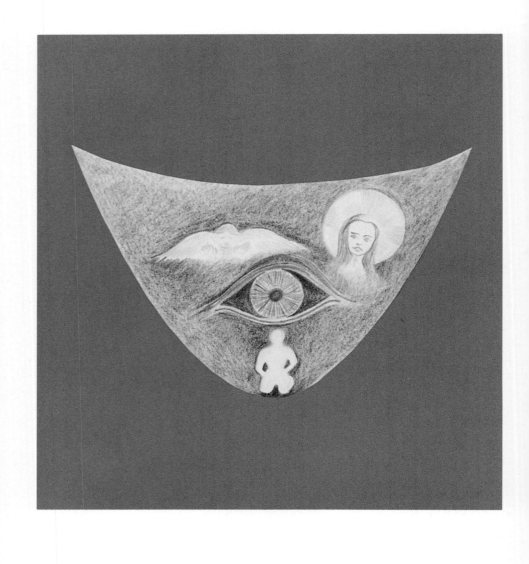

WORKSHEET NO. 7

Working with violet. You will need for this session a piece of amethyst.

1 Read the meaning of the colour violet.   Page 123

2 Start with a simple relaxation.   Page 24

3 Perform three rounds of Surya Namaskara.
Either visualise the relevant chakra or intone
the mantras belonging to the chakras.   Page 31

4 *ASANAS* Whilst holding these postures,
           bring your awareness into the relevant
           chakra and try to visualise the colour
           which radiates from it.

     a) Bakasana (Crown centre)   Page 128
     b) Gomukhasana (Brow centre)   Page 115
     c) Ardha Chandrasana (Throat centre)   Page 109
     d) Parivrtta Trikonasana (Heart centre)   Page 94
     e) Bhujangasana (Solar plexus centre)   Page 78
     f) Ardha Salabhasana and Salabhasana
        (Sacral centre)   Pages 69, 68
     g) The Arm Leg Link (Base centre)   Page 53

5 Repeat Bakasana, visualising the colour violet
radiating from the crown centre.

6 Visualisation and awareness exercise on the
colour violet.   Page 124

7 Meditation with the colour violet.   Page 132

8 General Relaxation No. 2. During this relaxation
be aware of any changes or experiences
you may have had.   Page 27

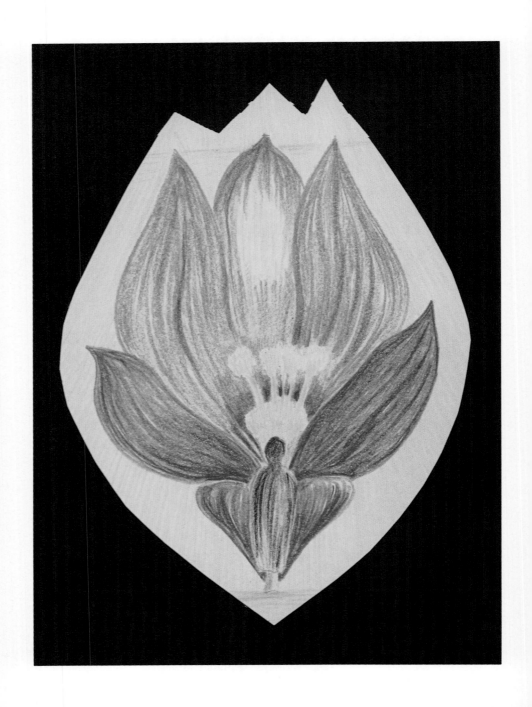

WORKSHEET NO. 8

Working with magenta. You will need a sheet of plain paper, a paintbrush, some magenta and white paint, and the picture on the back of this worksheet.

1 Read about the chakra of the higher self.   Page 171

2 Read the meaning of the colour magenta.   Page 172

3 Start with a simple relaxation.   Page 24

4 Perform three rounds of Surya Namaskara.
Either visualise the relevant chakra or intone
the mantras belonging to the chakras.   Page 31

5 *ASANAS* Whilst holding these postures,
bring your awareness into the relevant
chakra and try to visualise the colour
which radiates from it.

a) Bakasana (Crown centre) (Visualise the violet in this
centre, lifting up into a beautiful magenta.   Page 128
b) Halasana (Throat centre)   Page 105
c) Ardha Matsyendrasana (Brow centre)   Page 118
d) Parivrtta Trikonasana (Heart centre)   Page 94
e) Bhujangasana (Solar plexus centre)   Page 78
f) Ardha Salabhasana and Salabhasana
(Sacral centre)   Pages 69, 68
g) The Knee Lock (Base centre)   Page 50

6 Repeat Bakasana, visualising the violet lifting
up into a beautiful magenta.

7 Visualisation and awareness exercise on
the colour magenta. Use the picture on the
back of this worksheet.   Page 174

8 Meditation with the colour magenta.   Page 173

9 Relaxation and awareness exercise to balance
and energise the seven chakras.   Page 136

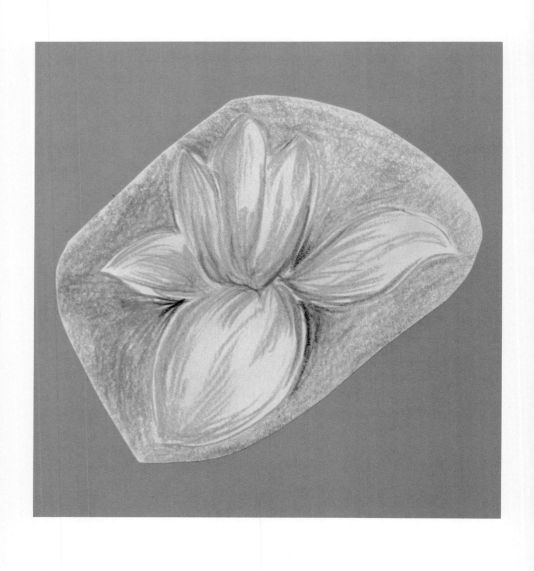

WORKSHEET NO. 9

Working with green. You will need for this session a place where there is green grass.

1 Read the meaning of the colour green.   Page 85

2 Start with a simple relaxation.   Page 24

3 Perform two rounds of Chandra Namaskara
(use as an awareness and warming up
exercise).   Page 144

4 *ASANAS* Whilst holding these postures,
           bring your awareness into the relevant
           chakra and try to visualise the colour
           which radiates from it.

    a) Bakasana (Crown centre)   Page 128
    b) Halasana (Throat centre)   Page 105
    c) Gomukhasana (Brow centre)   Page 115
    d) Matsyasana (If you are unable to sit in
       full lotus, practise the variations.)
       (Heart centre)   Page 88
    e) Ustrasana (Solar plexus centre)   Page 77
    f) Supta Virasana (Sacral centre)   Page 68
    g) Garudasana (Base centre)   Page 52

5 Repeat Matsyasana, visualising the colour
green radiating from the heart centre.

6 Visualisation and awareness exercise on green
(No. 2)   Page 87

7 Meditation from the heart chakra.   Page 96

8 General Relaxation No. 3. During this relaxation, be
aware of any changes or experiences you may have
had.   Page 28

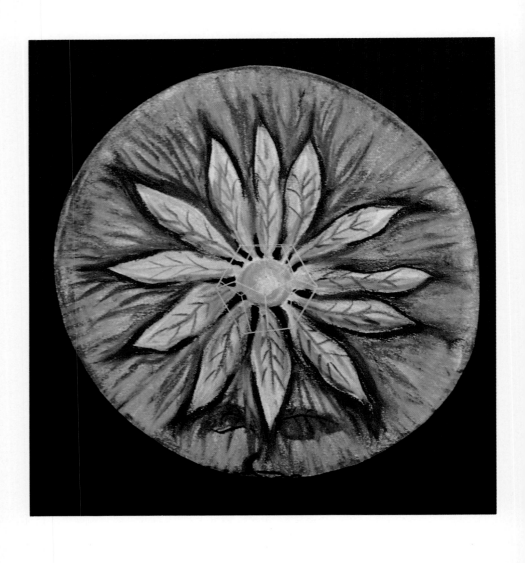

WORKSHEET NO. 10

Working with red. You will need for this session the picture of the Muladhara chakra, which is on the back of this worksheet.

1 Read the meaning of the colour red.   Page 46

2 Start with a simple relaxation.   Page 24

3 Perform two rounds of Chandra Namaskara (use as an awareness and warming up exercise).   Page 144

5 *ASANAS* Whilst holding these postures bring your awareness into the relevant chakra and try to visualise the colour which radiates from it.

a) Supported Head Balance (Read pages 129 and 130 before practising this.)
(Crown centre)   Page 129
b) Halasana (Throat centre)   Page 105
c) Gomukhasana (Brow centre)   Page 115
d) Simhasana or Matsyasana
(Heart centre)   Page 89 or 88
e) Ustrasana (Solar plexus centre)   Page 77
f) Supta Vajrasana (Sacral centre)   Page 67
g) Garudasana (Base centre)   Page 52

5 Repeat Garudasana, visualising red flowing from the base centre.

6 Visualisation and awareness exercise on red. Use the drawing of the Mulhadhara chakra which is on the back of this worksheet.   Page 48

7 Meditation with the colour red.   Page 57

8 General Relaxation No. 3. During this relaxation, be aware of any changes which may have taken place or experiences you may have had.   Page 28

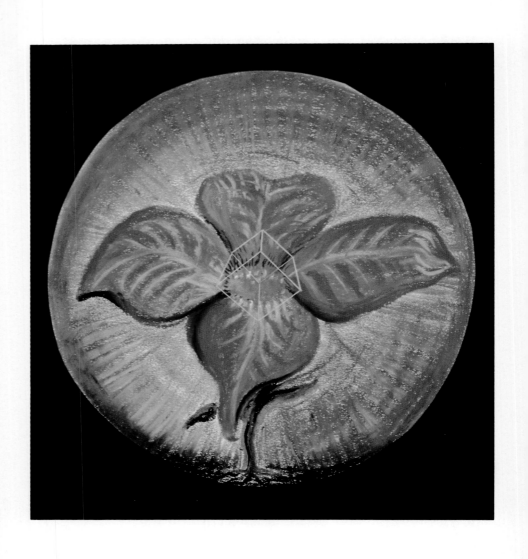

WORKSHEET NO. 11

Working with blue. You will need for this session a piece of blue material, either silk or cotton, which is 2 metres long and 1 metre wide.

1 Read the meaning of the colour blue.   Page 102

2 Start with a simple relaxation.   Page 24

3 Perform two rounds of Chandra Namaskara
  (use as an awareness and warming up
  exercise).   Page 144

4 *ASANAS* Whilst holding these postures
           bring your awareness into the relevant
           chakra and try to visualise the colour
           which radiates from it.

  a) Supported Head Balance (Read pages 129
     and 130 before practising this.)
     (Crown centre)   Page 129
  b) Halasana (Throat centre)   Page 105
  c) Ardha Matsyendrasana (Brow centre)   Page 118
  d) Baddha Padmasana (Heart centre)   Page 93
  e) Uttana Mayurasana (Solar plexus centre)   Page 80
  f) Padangusthasana (Sacral centre)   Page 66
  g) Ardha Navasana 1 (Base centre)   Page 50

5 Repeat Halasana, visualising the colour blue
  radiating from the throat centre.

6 Visualisation and awareness exercise on blue.
  Follow the instructions on page 103, but use
  blue material instead of yellow.   Page 103

7 Meditation on the colour blue.   Page 110

8 General Relaxation No. 3. During this relaxation,
  be aware of any changes which may have
  taken place or experiences you may have had.   Page 28

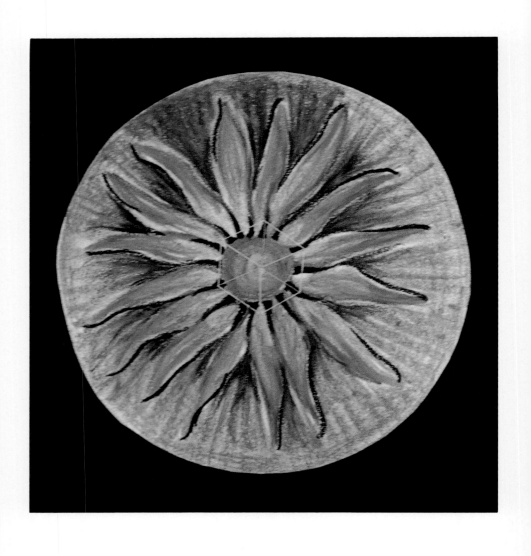

WORKSHEET NO. 12

Working with white. You will need for this session the picture on the back of this worksheet.

1 Read the meaning of the higher chakra of consciousness — white.   Page 174

2 Start with a simple relaxation.   Page 24

3 Perform two rounds of Chandra Namaskara.   Page 144

4 *ASANAS* Whilst holding these postures bring your awareness into the relevant chakra and try to visualise the colour which radiates from it.

   a) Sirasana. (For those who are unable to do Sirasana, practise one of the other postures which activate this chakra.) Whilst holding this posture, visualise the violet from the crown chakra lifting up into magenta and then into the pure white of God consciousness.   Page 129

   b) Sarvangasana or Halasana
     (Throat centre)   Page 107 or 105

   c) Ardha Matsyendrasana (Brow centre)   Page 118

   d) Baddha Padmasana (Heart centre)   Page 93

   e) Uttana Mayurasana (Solar plexus centre)   Page 80

   f) Padangusthasana (Sacral centre)   Page 66

   g) Ardha Navasana 2 (Base centre)   Page 51

5 Repeat Sirasana, as in 4a above.

6 Visualisation and awareness exercise on white. Page 176

7 Meditation on the colour white.   Page 175

8 General Relaxation No. 3. During this relaxation, be aware of any changes which may have taken place or experiences you may have had.   Page 28

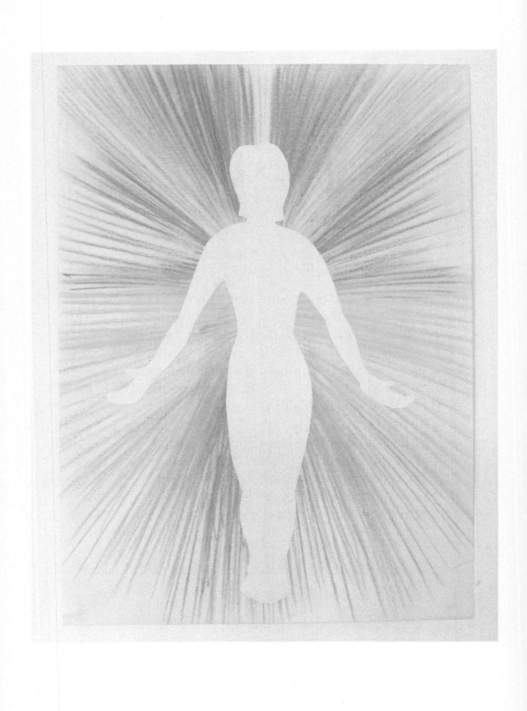

WORKSHEET NO. 13

Working with orange. For this session you will need a piece of carnelian.

1 Read the meaning of the colour orange.   Page 60

2 Start with a simple relaxation.   Page 24

3 Perform three rounds of Chandra Namaskara,
  Visualise the relevant chakra with each asana. Page 144

4 *ASANAS* Whilst holding these postures,
          bring your awareness into the relevant
          chakra and try to visualise the colour
          which radiates from it.

   a) Sirasana (For those who are unable to do
      Sirasana, practise one of the other postures
      which activate this chakra.)
      (Crown centre)   Page 129
   b) Sarvangasana (Throat centre)   Page 107
   c) Nataraja Asana (Brow centre)   Page 116
   d) Parivrtta Trikonasana (Heart centre)   Page 94
   e) Bhujangasana and Dhanurasana
      (Solar plexus centre)   Page 78, 79
   f) Salabhasana and Dhanurasana (Sacral and
      solar plexus centres)   Page 68, 79
   g) Yoga Mudrasana (Base centre)   Page 55

5 Repeat Salabhasana. Visualise the colour
  orange radiating from the sacral centre.

6 Visualisation and awareness exercise on orange. Page 61

7 Meditation with the colour orange.   Page 71

8 General Relaxation No. 1. During this
  relaxation, be aware of any changes which
  may have taken place or experiences you
  may have had.   Page 24

217

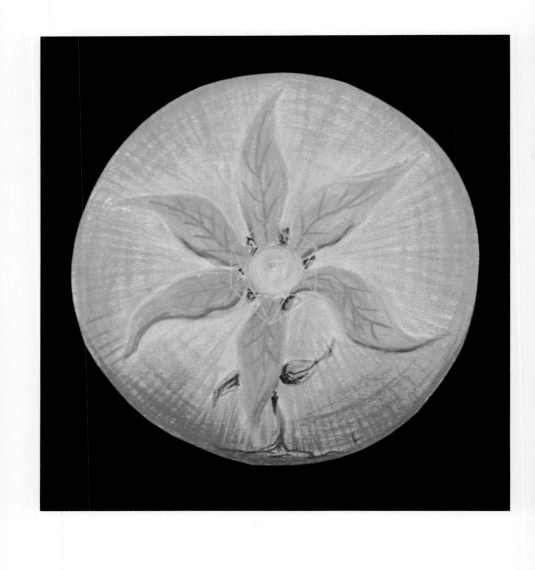

WORKSHEET NO. 14

Working with violet. For this session you will need a piece of amethyst.

1 Read the meaning of the colour violet. Page 123

2 Start with a simple relaxation. Page 24

3 Perform three rounds of Chandra Namaskara. Visualise the relevant chakra with each position. Page 144

4 *ASANAS* Whilst holding these postures, bring your awareness into the relevant chakra and try to visualise the colour which radiates from it.

a) Sirasana (For those who are unable to do Sirasana, practise one of the other postures which activate this chakra.) (Crown centre) Page 129
b) Sarvangasana (Throat centre) Page 107
c) Nataraja Asana (Brow centre) Page 116
d) Matsyasana (Heart centre) Page 88
e) Bhujangasana and Dhanurasana (Solar plexus centre) Pages 78, 79
f) Salabhasana and Dhanurasana (Sacral and solar plexus centre) Pages 68, 79
g) Yoga Mudrasana (Base centre) Page 55

5 Repeat Sirasana, visualising violet radiating from the crown chakra.

6 Visualisation and awareness exercise on violet. Page 124

7 Meditation on the colour violet (No. 2). Page 134

8 General Relaxation No. 1. During this relaxation, be aware of any changes which may have taken place or experiences you may have had. Page 24

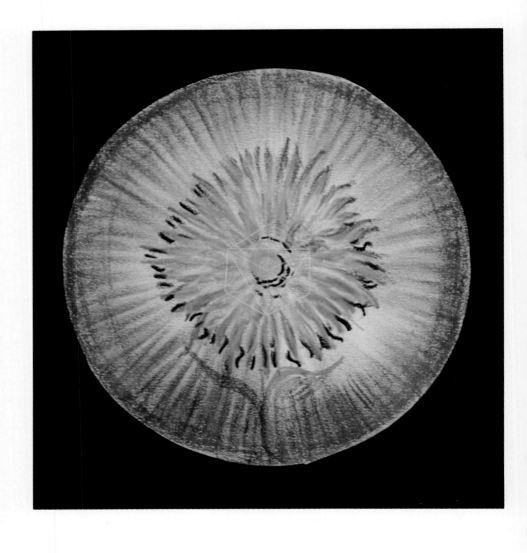

WORKSHEET NO. 15

Working with yellow. You will need for this session the picture of the Manipura chakra, which is on the back of this worksheet.

1 Read the meaning of the colour yellow. Page 74

2 Start with a simple relaxation. Page 24

3 Perform 3 rounds of Surya or Chandra Namaskara, as an awareness exercise, a visualisation of the chakras or intoning the mantras. Pages 31 or 144

4 *ASANAS* Whilst holding these postures, bring your awareness into the relevant chakra visualising the colour which radiates from it.

a) Salamba Sirasana (Crown centre) Page 131
b) Sarvangasana or Padma Sarvangasana (Throat centre) Page 107 or 108
c) Hanumanasana (Brow centre) Page 117
d) Simhasana or Virabhadrasana 1 and 2 (Heart centre) Page 89 or 91
e) Urdhva Dhanurasana or Uttana Mayurasana (Solar plexus centre) Page 81 or 80
f) Kurmasana (Sacral centre) Page 70
g) Padmasana or Yoga Mudrasana (Base centre) Page 54 or 55

5 Repeat either Urdhva Dhanurasana or Uttana Mayurasana, visualising yellow radiating from the solar plexus chakra.

6 Visualisation and awareness exercise on yellow. Use the drawing on the back of this worksheet. Page 75

7 Meditation with the colour yellow. Page 82

8 General Relaxation No. 1. Page 24

221

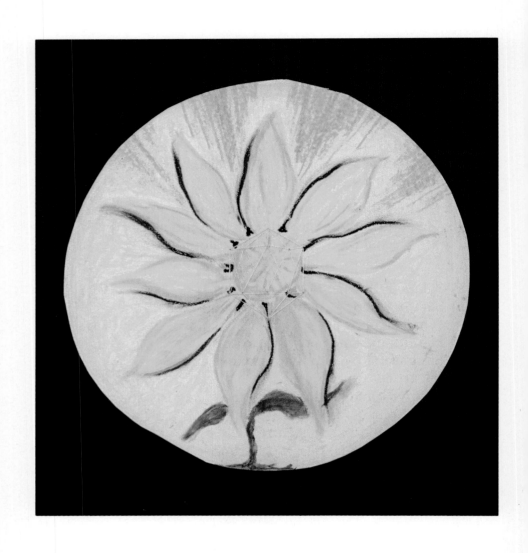

WORKSHEET NO. 16

Working with magenta. For this session you will need the picture of the Sahasrara yantra, on the back of this worksheet.

1 Read about the chakra of the higher self.   Page 171

2 Read about the meaning of magenta.   Page 172

3 Start with a simple relaxation.   Page 24

4 Perform three rounds of either Surya or Chandra Namaskara. Visualise the relevant chakra with each position.   Page 31 or 144

5 *ASANAS* Whilst holding these postures, bring your awareness into the relevant chakra and try to visualise the colour which radiates from it.

   a) Salamba Sirasana (Crown centre)   Page 131
   b) Sarvangasana going into Halasana
      (Throat centre)   Pages 107, 105
   c) Hanumanasana (Brow centre)   Page 117
   d) Gupta Padmasana or Virabhadrasana
      1 and 2 (Heart centre)   Page 90 or 91
   e) Urdhva Dhanurasana or Uttana Mayurasana
      (Solar plexus centre)   Page 81 or 80
   f) Kurmasana (Sacral centre)   Page 70
   g) Padmasana (Base centre)   Page 54

6 Repeat Salamba Sirasana and visualise the violet from this chakra lifting up into a magenta.

7 Visualisation and awareness exercise on magenta. Follow the instructions on page 174 but use the drawing of the Sahasrara yantra.   Page 174

8 Chakra meditation.   Page 140

9 General Relaxation.   Page 24

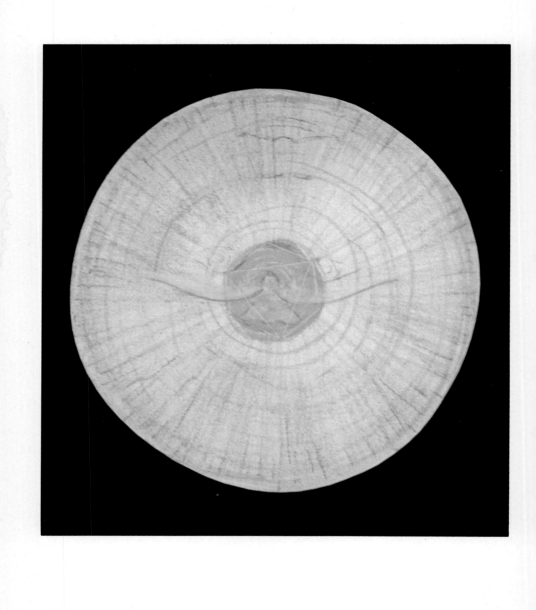